MEDICAL BOARDS STEP 1
made ridiculously simple

Andreas Carl, M.D., Ph.D.
Adjunct Assistant Professor
University of Nevada Reno
School of Medicine
Department of Physiology and Cell Biology
Reno, NV 89557-0046

MedMaster, Inc., Miami

Published by
MedMaster, Inc.
P.O. Box 640028
Miami, FL 33164

For Dr. Anna Ivanenko.

This project would not have been possible without her
encouragement and enthusiasm.

INTRODUCTION

What kind of score you will get on the USMLE Step 1 exam not only depends on how hard you study, but also on what you study. Obviously, if you study what they ask, you will achieve a very high score. I have prepared this manuscript in order to help you maximizing your efforts. The material has been selected based on many years of teaching basic medical sciences to medical students and my own experience taking the USMLE Step 1. Recently there have been significant changes in the USMLE format and content and I wish to thank the many students whose input has allowed me to keep this book current and relevant for the USMLE exam.

Please visit my web-site to share your experiences with other students:

http://www.usmle.net

If you are about to take the exam or just took it, you can contact me via e-mail:

Andreas_Carl@usmle.net

THE USMLE STEP 1 EXAM HAS BECOME SO CLINICAL IN NATURE, SHOULD I STUDY INTERNAL MEDICINE?

You will find that most exam questions are "wrapped" in a clinical case presentation, but in the end you still need to know the basic sciences in order to answer the questions. It is NOT necessary to know internal medicine to pass this exam (although it wouldn't hurt). Practically what this means for your test preparation is that you should focus on areas of basic science that have clear relevance to clinical medicine since these are much more likely to be made into a "case vignette" than esoteric science facts. For this reason I have greatly increased the number of clinical comments and explanations throughout this book.

WHAT ARE HIGH-YIELD FACTS?

You need to know that what may be of high yield in one year could very well be of low yield the next year. There are some clear trends over the year (for example the de-emphasis of gross anatomy) but even these may change next time around. Other "trends" are much more short lived events (for example the surprisingly small number of micro-biology questions on the Spring 1998 exam). In other words, you cannot rely on high-yield facts alone. I have listed student's impressions from previous exams on my web-site, so you might get a feel for important trends:

http://www.usmle.net/1996.html
http://www.usmle.net/1997.html
http://www.usmle.net/1998.html

WHY THE CHART FORMAT?

I have arranged all material in this book in the form of charts. This allows a logical arrangement of basic science facts which can easily be build upon rather than a random collection of materials. Studying in such systematic fashion lets you avoid the "high-yield trap". I have chosen the chart- format in order to provide the maximum amount of information with the minimum amount of words. By concentrating on key associations you will certainly improve your performance in "multiple choice situations".

WHAT THIS BOOK IS NOT:

Medical Boards Step 1 Made Ridiculously Simple is not a text book. I have tried to be clear and comprehensive but brief. You will find most of the material very simplified, perhaps oversimplified and sometimes you may find it necessary to consult your textbooks, in order to make sense out of it. As you become familiar with the material, you should be able to read through these tables within a few hours and still maintain a relaxed state of mind - now you are ready to take the USMLE Step 1 exam!

HOW TO USE THIS BOOK?

This book is best used side by side with your other text and review books. You can "personalize" the charts by adding information that appears important or interesting to you. **The logical arrangement of basic science facts in charts will make it very easy to review all USMLE subjects just a few days before the exam**. I recommend reviewing the tables many times until they become boring. This is a good sign - meaning you recognize the stuff. It's NOT necessary to be able to actively reproduce the material given here, as long as you recognize the key associations in a "multiple choice situation".

A few words about selection of this material: You will find Anatomy, Social Sciences and Physiology slightly underrepresented and Pathology somewhat over-represented here. Anatomy has been kept short because a) it's highly visual, you profit more by looking at the pictures in an atlas, rather than reading words, b) there have been only few Gross Anatomy questions on recent USMLE Step 1 exams. Social Sciences and Physiology are underrepresented because they are conceptual sciences and contain a smaller amount of hard core facts. I have overemphasized Pathology somewhat, because I believe it is the most useful of the basic sciences for your future career and will be an invaluable help for studying of Internal Medicine in the 3rd and 4th years of Medical School.

I wish to thank Steve Goldberg for the cartoons. Figures 4.23-4.32 were modified and reproduced with permission from Smith, L.H. and Thier, S.O. *Pathophysiology - The Biological Principles of Disease*. W.D. Saunders Co., 1985.

I hope that this text will help your preparation for the USMLE Step 1 and would appreciate any comments about the selection and presentation of this material you might have. Good luck!

```
www.usmle.net
• latest trends on the USMLE
• new updates
• hot links
```

PATHOLOGY

- This should be the center piece of your studies, it's also the most valuable for your future practice.

- Both Rubin and Farber's Pathology (16) and Robbins-Cotran (14) are excellent text books but too long for review. If you have used them during your class you may want to review the pictures and highlighted texts. The Board Review Series Pathology book by Schneider and Szanto (17) is highly recommended.

- Spend a day just looking at pictures, until you can distinguish a papillary thyroid carcinoma from a follicular one (with closed eyes, in the middle of the night and blind - just kidding).

- If you are ambitious, go over Compton's Review Questions (15). These are very difficult! If you get about 50% right, you should do very well on the Boards.

MICROBIOLOGY

- Just study them bug by bug, Levinson-Jawetz (13) is an excellent text.

- Also check out *Clinical Microbiology Made Ridiculously Simple* (6). This book contains over 200 cartoons which makes microbiology actually fun.

- Know all the details, structure/function of the HIV virus. Study therapy of AIDS related infectious diseases.

- If you have time to spare, read "Immunology" from the NMS series (12). There are many questions on the exam, and this book covers it all.

PHARMACOLOGY

- Harvey-Champe (19) is "dead-on". If you know this book, you should get close to 100% right.

- *Clinical Pharmacology Made Ridiculously Simple* (8) contains a large number of tables comparing drugs side by side. Very complete! Excellent review, not just for the Boards but also for later.

- I found flash cards very useful. Make two sets: one for drug names versus mechanism of action and/or indication, and one set for drug names versus side effects.

BIOCHEMISTRY

- Champe-Harvey (2) is "dead-on". If you know this book, you should get close to 100% right.

- In case you got lost, I recommend *Clinical Biochemistry Made Ridiculously Simple* (5) for a quick overview of the wondrous and amazing Land of Biochemistry.

ANATOMY

- Don't spend too much time on this subject. Best preparation is to look at pictures, including plenty of cross sections (CT or MRI scans) of the body.

- Read *Clinical Anatomy Made Ridiculously Simple* (4), but even this may be overkill.

- Read *Clinical Neuroanatomy Made Ridiculously Simple* (7). Read this one twice!

- Make sure you know basic Embryology to get some easy points.

PHYSIOLOGY

- A difficult subject because you cannot memorize it. Even if you knew your Ganong (21) or Guyton (24), you may not be able to answer all questions. I very much like the *Color Atlas of Physiology* by Despopoulos and Silbernagel (9) for quick review.

- Concentrate on kidneys, heart and lungs!

- A recent trend on the USMLE is receptors, signal transduction mechanisms and molecular biology of the cell.

- Make sure you can calculate renal clearance without getting a panic attack!

SOCIAL SCIENCES

- Don't waste too much time here, but read *USMLE Behavioral Science Made Ridiculously Simple* (25). Some things you need to know very well are:

- Differences between normal grief reaction and adjustment disorders, neuroses and psychoses, dementia and delirium.
- Defense mechanisms.
- Sensitivity / Specificity / Negative predictive value etc. It's not enough to memorize what to divide by what, you need to understand the meaning of these.
- Design of clinical trials.
- Signs of child abuse.

PRACTICE QUESTIONS

- You will find the real exam very different from any collection of multiple choice questions or practice tests currently on the market. The real exam is more clinical in nature and questions tend to be longer. Don't panic - everyone is "in the same boat". There are retired board questions, but remember: they are retired for a reason! I found the *Pretest Questions* slightly more difficult than the actual board exam. The Appleton & Lange (1) and NMS questions (22) are a bit easier. Practice as many questions as possible.

- Don't use questions to "test" yourself. Don't be concerned about how many percent you get right. Mark all questions you get wrong with a pen, identify your areas of weakness and concentrate your studies on these. Later review just the questions you got wrong the first time and see how much you have learned.

- Don't practice multiple choice questions the week before the exam. You will get tired, bored and frustrated. Negative feelings might carry over to the exam day.

TEST TAKING STRATEGIES

- Don't study any new material the day before the exam. It's more important to be well rested.

- If you can't even guess a question, choose either the longest answer or the one that is most similar to other choices. Then move on. Don't be upset, this happens a lot and is quite normal. If you have the feeling you might be able to answer it if you could only think hard enough, skip it and come back to it if time allows.

- Make sure you time yourself very well. I found it useful to answer questions in blocks of 15. This saves a little time and you get breaks marking the sheet.

- Avoid burnout. Make a fresh start with each booklet, no matter how well or badly you think you did the previous one.

ADVICE FOR FOREIGN MEDICAL GRADUATES

- It's especially important to get a good score the first time around since it has become more and more difficult for foreign medical graduates to get into a Residency program.

- Only 50% of foreign medical graduates pass on first attempt, compared to 95% of US and Canadian medical students. A major reason for this difference is language comprehension.

- Questions on the USMLE have become exceedingly long and you may struggle finishing in time. Practice as many questions as you can (at least 1,000). Make sure to practice some under "real-time" conditions: try to finish 180 questions in 2½ hours without a break.

- It is useful to read the last sentence of each question first, then take a quick glance (no more!) at the answer choices, then go back and read the text of the question very selectively.

REFERENCES

1. A&L's Review for the USMLE Step 1, T.K. Barton, Appleton & Lange
2. Biochemistry, Champe & Harvey, Lippincott
3. Biochemistry, Stryer, Freeman
4. Clinical Anatomy Made Ridiculously Simple, S.Goldberg, MedMaster
5. Clinical Biochemistry Made Ridiculously Simple, S.Goldberg, MedMaster
6. Clinical Microbiology Made Ridiculously Simple, Gladwin & Trattler, MedMaster
7. Clinical Neuroanatomy Made Ridiculously Simple, S.Goldberg, MedMaster
8. Clinical Pharmacology Made Ridiculously Simple, J. Olson, MedMaster
9. Color-Atlas of Physiology, Despopoulos & Silbernagl, Thieme
10. Comprehensive Textbook of Psychiatry, Kaplan, Williams & Wilkin
11. Drug Evaluations, American Medical Association
12. Immunology, R.Hyde, Harwal Publishing
13. Medical Microbiology & Immunology, Levinson-Jawetz, Appleton & Lange
14. Pathologic Basis of Disease, Robbins & Cotran, Saunders
15. Pathologic Basis of Disease - Selfassessment and Review, Saunders
16. Pathology, Rubin & Farber, Lippincott
17. Pathology, Schneider & Szanto, Board Review Series, Williams & Wilkin
18. Pharmacologic Basis of Therapeutics, Goodman & Gilman, Macmillan
19. Pharmacology, Harvey & Champe, Lippincott
20. Physiological Basis of Medical Practice, J.B.West, Williams & Wilkin
21. Review of Medical Physiology, W.F. Ganong, Appleton & Lange
22. Review for USMLE Step 1, NMS, Williams & Wilkin
23. Sherris Medical Microbiology, K.J. Ryan, Appleton & Lange
24. Textbook of Medical Physiology, Guyton & Hall, Saunders
25. USMLE Behavioral Science Made Ridiculously Simple, F. Sierles, MedMaster

ℭℨℭℨℭℨℭℨℭℨℭℨℭℨℭℨℭℨℭℨℭℨℭℨℭℨℭℨℭℨℭℨ

WHAT'S NEXT ?

If you liked this book and passed the USMLE Step 1 exam: Keep it!

You will need Chapters 1-3 (Pathology, Microbiology and Pharmacology) for a lightening fast review just prior to taking the Step 2 exam. My book *Medical Boards Step 2 Made Ridiculously Simple* will help you prepare for this exam but I have not repeated this information in the Step 2 book. It's always best to do your review from books and materials you already have mastered once.

CONTENTS

1. **PATHOLOGY** 1
   General Pathology 2
   Organ Pathology 18

2. **MICROBIOLOGY** 83
   General Microbiology 84
   Bacteria 90
   Viruses 107
   Fungi & Parasites 114

3. **PHARMACOLOGY** 125

4. **BIOCHEMISTRY** 177

5. **ANATOMY** 227
   Embryology 228
   Gross Anatomy 233
   Neuroanatomy 251

6. **PHYSIOLOGY** 265

7. **SOCIAL SCIENCES** 303

8. **ABBREVIATIONS** 331

9. **INDEX** 333

TABLE OF CONTENTS

PATHOLOGY

GENERAL PATHOLOGY

1.1. Inflammation
1.2. Cytokines
1.3. Complement
1.4. Autoantibodies
1.5. Amyloid
1.6. Hypersensitivity
1.7. Oncogenes
1.8. Tumor suppressor genes
1.9. Tumor markers

1.10. Metastases
1.11. Genetics - Pedigrees
1.12. Autosomal recessive diseases
1.13. Autosomal dominant diseases
1.14. X-linked recessive diseases
1.15. Deletions
1.16. HLA
1.17. Most common causes

ORGAN PATHOLOGY

1.18. SLE
1.19. Systemic sclerosis
1.20. Sjögren's syndrome
1.21. Immunodeficiencies
1.22. Bleeding disorders
1.23. Hemolytic anemias
1.24. Other anemias
1.25. Red blood cells
1.26. Neutropenia
1.27. Leukocytosis
1.28. Leukemias
1.29. Lymphomas
1.30. Plasma cell neoplasias
1.31. Phlebothrombosis
1.32. Arteriosclerosis
1.33. Arteritis
1.34. Aneurysms
1.35. Heart sounds
1.36. Congenital heart defects
1.37. Ischemic heart disease
1.38. Myocardial infarction
1.39. Heart failure
1.40. Endocarditis

1.41. Pericarditis
1.42. Rheumatic heart disease
1.43. Obstructive lung diseases
1.44. Restrictive lung diseases
1.45. Pneumonia
1.46. Lung tumors
1.47. Glomerulonephritis I
1.48. Glomerulonephritis II
1.49. Urolithiasis
1.50. Venereal diseases
1.51. Testes tumors
1.52. Ovarian tumors
1.53. Endometrium
1.54. Placenta
1.55. Breast
1.56. Mouth
1.57. Esophageal diverticula
1.58. Gastritis
1.59. Gastroenteritis
1.60. Polyposis of colon
1.61. Inflammatory bowel disease
1.62. Malabsorption
1.63. Cholelithiasis

1.64. Carcinomas
1.65. Jaundice
1.66. Hepatitis
1.67. Hepatitis B serology
1.68. Toxic hepatitis
1.69. Cirrhosis
1.70. Liver carcinoma
1.71. Arthritis
1.72. Bones
1.73. Cartilage
1.74. Bone tumors
1.75. Muscular dystrophies
1.76. Brain tumors
1.77. CNS degeneration

1.78. Demyelinating diseases
1.79. Pituitary hyperfunction
1.80. Pituitary hypofunction
1.81. Adrenal adenomas / carcinomas
1.82. Thyroid
1.83. Thyroid tumors
1.84. Parathyroids
1.85. Diabetes mellitus
1.86. Multiple endocrine neoplasia
1.87. Skin cancer
1.88. Other skin diseases
1.89. Toxins

MICROBIOLOGY

GENERAL MICROBIOLOGY

2.1. Stains
2.2. Normal flora
2.3. Cell walls

2.4. Toxins
2.5. O_2-Requirements
2.6 Most common causes

BACTERIA

2.7. Staphylococci
2.8. Streptococci
2.9. Neisseria
2.10. Bacilli
2.11. Gram-positive bacilli
2.12. Clostridia
2.13. Enterobacteriaceae
2.14. More Enterobacteriaceae

2.15. Gram-negative bacilli (zoonotic)
2.16. Other gram-negative bacilli
2.17. Mycobacteria
2.18. Higher bacteria
2.19. Spirochetes
2.20. Chlamydia
2.21 Rickettsia

VIRUSES

2.22. DNA viruses
2.23. Herpes viruses
2.24. RNA viruses
2.25. ARBO viruses

2.26. Slow viral diseases of CNS
2.27. Prions
2.28. Retroviruses
2.29. HIV

FUNGI & PARASITES

2.30. Fungi
2.31. Fungal diseases
2.32. Malaria
2.33. Tissue protozoa

2.34. Intestinal protozoa
2.35. Trematodes (flukes)
2.36. Cestodes (tapeworms)
2.37 Nematodes (roundworms)

PHARMACOLOGY

3.1 Drug interactions
3.2. Bad combinations
3.3. Famous side effects
3.4. Antidotes
3.5. Antibiotics
3.6. Drugs of choice
3.7. Penicillins
3.8. Cephalosporins
3.9. Antiviral drugs
3.10. Antifungal drugs
3.11. Antiprotozoal drugs
3.12. AIDS
3.13. Inhibitors of translation
3.14. Inhibitors of replication
3.15. Inhibitors of transcription
3.16. Combination chemotherapy
3.17. NSAIDs
3.18. Gout
3.19. Antihypertensive drugs
3.20. Anti-angiotensins
3.21. Ergot alkaloids
3.22. Diuretics

3.23. Antianginal drugs
3.24. Platelet aggregation inhibitors
3.25. Anticoagulants
3.26. Antiarrhythmic drugs
3.27. Inotropic drugs
3.28. Asthma
3.29. Insulins
3.30. Sulfonylureas
3.31. Hyperlipidemias
3.32. Hyperlipidemia drugs
3.33. Peptic ulcers
3.34. Adrenergic drugs
3.35. Cholinesterase inhibitors
3.36. Direct cholinergic drugs
3.37. Antimuscarinic drugs
3.38. Antinicotinic drugs
3.39. Sex-hormones
3.40. Hallucinogens
3.41. Opioids
3.42. Antidepressants
3.43. Lithium

3.44. CNS stimulants
3.45. Anxiolytic drugs
3.46. Hypnotic drugs
3.47. Antihistamines
3.48. Anesthetics

3.49. Parkinson's disease
3.50. Neuroleptics
3.51. Antiepileptic drugs
3.52. Antiemetic drugs
3.53 Laxatives

BIOCHEMISTRY

4.1. Enzyme kinetics
4.2. Amino acids
4.3. Amino acid precursors
4.4. Amino acid disorders
4.5. Enzyme defects
4.6. Hexoses
4.7. Hexose kinases
4.8. Saccharides
4.9. Saccharide disorders
4.10. Enzyme defects
4.11. Glycogen storage diseases
4.12. Enzyme defects
4.13. Glycosaminoglycans
4.14. Fatty acids
4.15. Bile acids
4.16. Phospholipids
4.17. Sphingolipids
4.18. Sphingolipidoses
4.19. Enzyme defects
4.20. Porphyrias
4.21. Enzyme defects
4.22. Preferred fuels
4.23. Vitamins

4.24. ATP equivalents
4.25. Key enzymes - sugars
4.26. Key enzymes - fats
4.27. Key enzymes - others
4.28. Steroids
4.29. Adrenal gland
4.30. Testis (Leydig cells)
4.31. Peripheral metabolism
4.32. Ovary (Theca cells)
4.33. Ovary (Granulosa cells)
4.34. Peripheral metabolism
4.35. Corpus luteum
4.36. 17-α-hydroxylase deficiency
4.37. 21-α-hydroxylase deficiency
4.38. 11-β-hydroxylase
4.39. Endocrine control of metabolism
4.40. Nucleotides
4.41. Purines
4.42. Pyrimidines
4.43. Gene expression
4.44. Transcription
4.45 Replication

ANATOMY

EMBRYOLOGY

5.1.   Germ layers
5.2.   Fetal remnants
5.3.   Derivatives of branchial arches

5.4.   Pharyngeal pouches
5.5.   Urogenital development

GROSS ANATOMY

5.6.   The skull and its holes
5.7.   Eye
5.8.   Tongue
5.9.   Mandible
5.10. Larynx
5.11. Shoulder
5.12. Brachial plexus
5.13. Brachial nerve injuries
5.14. Elbow

5.15. Hip
5.16. Knee
5.17. Ankle
5.18. Mediastinum
5.19. Coronary arteries
5.20. Abdominal arteries
5.21. Peritoneum
5.22. Layers of spermatic cord
5.23   Ovary / testis

NEUROANATOMY

5.24. Cortex
5.25. Cerebral arteries
5.26. Transient ischemic attacks
5.27. Hypertensive hemorrhage
5.28. Cranial nerves
5.29. Parasympathetic ganglia
5.30. Basal ganglia

5.31. Thalamus
5.32. Brainstem syndromes
5.33. Medulla
5.34. Lower pons
5.35. Upper pons
5.36. Where is the lesion?
5.37   Key dermatomes

PHYSIOLOGY

6.1.   Six equations you really need
6.2.   Ion channels
6.3.   Transport
6.4.   Signal transduction
6.5.   Nerve fibers
6.6.   Touch receptors
6.7.   Accommodation
6.8.   Nystagmus
6.9.   Cochlea
6.10. Deafness
6.11. Autonomic nervous system
6.12. Muscarinic receptors
6.13. Adrenergic receptors
6.14. Control of heart beat
6.15. Control of muscle tone
6.16. Muscle types
6.17. Electromechanical coupling
6.18. Cardiac cycle
6.19. Lung volumes

6.20. Breathing patterns
6.21. Respiratory quotient
6.22. Acid base
6.23. Hemoglobins
6.24. Oxygen binding curve
6.25. Blood proteins
6.26. Circulation
6.27. Fetal circulation
6.28. Renal transport
6.29. Clearance
6.30. Volume regulation
6.31. Renin / Angiotensin
6.32. Intestinal absorption
6.33. Stomach
6.34. Gastrointestinal hormones
6.35. Adrenal hormones
6.36. Insulin
6.37   Gonadotrope hormones

SOCIAL SCIENCES

PSYCHOLOGY

7.1.   Motor development
7.2.   Psychological development
7.3.   IQ tests
7.4.   Conditioning

7.5.   Defense mechanisms
7.6.   Sleep stages
7.7.   Suicide
7.8.   Stages of dying

PSYCHOPATHOLOGY

7.9.   Neurotransmitters
7.10. Grief & Depression
7.11. Delirium & Dementia
7.12. Personality types
7.13. Anxiety disorders

7.14. Somatoform disorders
7.15. Psychoses
7.16. Epilepsy
7.17. Drug abuse
7.18. Child abuse

STATISTICS

7.19. Definitions
7.20. Sensitivity
7.21. Specificity
7.22. Positive predictive value
7.23. Negative predictive value
7.24. Cancer statistics (USA)

7.25. Randomized clinical trial
7.26. Observational cohort
7.27. Case control study
7.28. Cross sectional survey
7.29   Legal issues

PATHOLOGY

Part A : General Pathology

1.1.) INFLAMMATION

> red - tender - warm - swollen

ACUTE INFLAMMATION:
- increased blood flow
- increased vascular permeability
- emigration of leukocytes

MEDIATORS OF INFLAMMATION:

fever	IL-1, prostaglandins
vasodilatation	nitric oxide
	prostaglandins
exudation	histamine, bradykinin
chemotaxis	complement C5a, IL-8
phagocytosis	complement C3b (opsonin)
pain	prostaglandins, bradykinin

Note how inhibitors of prostaglandin synthesis (e.g. aspirin) alleviate many symptoms of inflammation (fever, swelling, pain) but not necessarily the inflammatory process itself!

1.2.) CYTOKINES

* most cytokines have a wide spectrum of effects
* many cytokines are produced by several cell types

MAIN FUNCTIONS OF CYTOKINES:

proinflammatory (produced by phagocytes)	IL-1, IL-8, TNF-α
activators of lymphocytes	IL-2, IL-4, IL-5
hematopoiesis	stem cell factor (c-kit ligand) colony stimulating factors

It is an almost hopeless task to list all interactions between cells during an inflammatory process. Some of the major ones you may want to know:

antigen presenting cell (macrophages)	->	**IL-1**	->	**CD4 helper T cell**
CD4 helper T cell	->	**IL-2**	->	**natural killer cells, cytotoxic T cells**
CD4 helper cell	->	**INF-γ**	->	**monocytes**
T cells	->	**IL-2, 4, 5**	->	**B cells**
monocytes	->	**IL-6, 8**	->	**B cells**

3

MAJOR CYTOKINES:

	produced by:	action:
α-interferon	leukocytes	antiviral induces MHC-I
β-interferon	fibroblasts	antiviral
γ-interferon	T cells	activates macrophages induces MHC-II
TNF	macrophages	fever, cachexia etc.
IL-1	macrophages	fever
IL-2, IL-3, IL-4, IL-5	T cells	activate many other cells
IL-6	macrophages fibroblasts	activates B cells
IL-7	bone marrow cells	proliferation of B and T cells
PDGF	platelets endothelial cells	proliferation of vascular smooth muscle cells

1.3.) <u>COMPLEMENT</u>

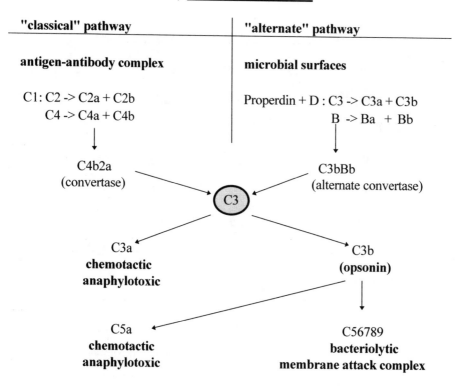

"classical" pathway	"alternate" pathway
antigen-antibody complex	microbial surfaces

"classical" pathway

C1: C2 -> C2a + C2b
    C4 -> C4a + C4b

C4b2a
(convertase)

"alternate" pathway

Properdin + D : C3 -> C3a + C3b
    B -> Ba + Bb

C3bBb
(alternate convertase)

C3

C3a
chemotactic
anaphylotoxic

C3b
(opsonin)

C5a
chemotactic
anaphylotoxic

C56789
bacteriolytic
membrane attack complex

 Activation of the alternate pathway does not require specific antibodies.

1.4.) AUTOANTIBODIES

rheumatoid arthritis	anti-IgG (rheumatoid factor)
systemic lupus	anti-nuclear antibodies (ANA)
drug induced lupus	anti-histone
CREST	anti-centromere
myasthenia gravis	anti-ACh receptor
Graves' disease	anti-TSH receptor
Hashimoto's thyroiditis	anti-microsomal
Wegener's granulomatosis	anti-neutrophil cytoplasm (ANCA)
primary biliary cirrhosis	anti-mitochondrial
celiac sprue	anti-gliadin
Goodpasture's syndrome	anti glomerular basement membrane

1.5.) AMYLOID

- *amorphous, eosinophilic extracellular substance*
- *consists of fibril protein and glycoprotein*
- *Congo-Red stain -> green birefringence under polarizing microscope*
- *this distinguishes amyloid from other hyaline deposits (collagen, fibrin)*

MAJOR FORMS OF AMYLOID:

AL:	Amyloid light chains	a/w multiple myeloma
AA:	Amyloid associated protein	a/w chronic inflammation and aging

---

1.6.) HYPERSENSITIVITY

	mediators	signs & symptoms	examples
Type I	**IgE** mast cells basophils	urticaria erythema bronchiole constr. laryngeal edema shock, death	**asthma** hay fever eczema
Type II	**IgM, IgG** antibody dependent cell mediated cytotoxicity	hemolysis	**transfusion reaction** drug reactions erythroblastosis fetalis autoimmune diseases
Type III	**IgM, IgG** immune complexes	urticaria lymphadenopathy arthritis vasculitis glomerulonephritis	**serum sickness** Arthus reaction
Type IV	"delayed hypersensitivity" **T cell** mediated (memory cells)	erythema with induration	**tuberculin reaction**

- Serum sickness: nowadays mostly caused by drugs
- Arthus reaction: edema and necrosis following intradermal injection of drugs

	Transplant rejection:
hyperacute:	due to preformed antibodies
acute:	involves type I and type IV mechanisms

1.7.) ONCOGENES

v-onc: oncogenes found in viruses.
c-onc: (protooncogene) cellular DNA that resembles viral oncogenes.
When activated will cause malignancy.

	gene product	disease
c-myc	transcription factor	Burkitt lymphoma
c-abl	tyrosine kinase	CML
bcl-2	inhibits apoptosis	Non-Hodgkin lymphoma
ras	G protein	colon carcinoma

1.8.) TUMOR SUPPRESSOR GENES

Loss of specific suppressor genes promotes malignancy.

	disease
RB1	retinoblastoma
BRCA-1	breast cancer ovarian cancer
p53	breast carcinoma colon carcinoma bronchial carcinomas

1.9.) <u>TUMOR MARKERS</u>

CEA	- **adenocarcinomas** (colon, pancreas, lung)
alpha-fetoprotein	- **hepatoma** - twin pregnancy - anencephalus
PSA	- **prostate carcinoma** - more sensitive than acid phosphatase
acid phosphatase	- **prostate carcinoma**
alkaline phosphatase	- **metastases to bones** - **obstructive biliary disease** - Paget's disease

 Tumor markers are mainly used for follow-up after treatment, not for screening an asymptomatic population.

1.10.) <u>METASTASES</u>

	most common primary site
brain	lung > breast
bone	breast > lung
liver	colon > stomach > pancreas

1.11.) GENETICS - PEDIGREES

AUTOSOMAL DOMINANT:

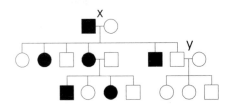

X: Sick person marries healthy one: 50% of children will be sick
                                                              males and females have equal risk
Y: Healthy child marries healthy persons: 100% normal offspring

Every sick person has at least one sick parent!

AUTOSOMAL RECESSIVE:

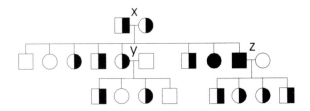

X: If two heterozygotes marry: 25% children will be normal
                                                        50% children will be heterozygous
                                                        25% children will be sick

Y: Heterozygote marries healthy: 50% children will be normal
                                                        50% children will be heterozygous
                                                          0% children will be sick

Z: Homozygote marries healthy: 100% children will be heterozygous

X-LINKED RECESSIVE:

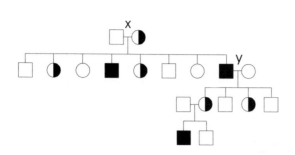

X: Carrier marries healthy male: *50% sons will be sick*
                                       50% sons will be healthy
                                       100% daughters will be healthy
                                       50% daughters will be carriers

Y: Sick male marries healthy female: *all sons will be healthy*
                                         all daughters will be carriers

Disease tends to skip generations!
Male to male transmission of disease rules out X-linked disease!

☐ healthy male
○ healthy female
■ sick male
● sick female
◑ heterozygote (carrier)

1.12.) <u>AUTOSOMAL RECESSIVE DISEASES</u>

cystic fibrosis	pulmonary infections, chronic pancreatitis
phenylketonuria	fair skin, blue eyes, mental retardation if untreated
albinism	sunburn, squamous carcinoma of skin
α1-antitrypsin deficiency	COPD, liver cirrhosis
thalassemias, sickle cell anemias	anemia
glycogen storage diseases	affect liver, muscles, heart (plus hypoglycemia in some)
mucopolysaccharidoses (except Hunter's)	*lysosomal storage disease* facial deformities, mental and physical retardation
sphingolipidoses (except Fabry's)	*lysosomal storage disease* hepatomegaly, splenomegaly etc.
polycystic renal disease (infant type)	kidney failure
hemochromatosis	liver cirrhosis, diabetes, cardiac failure
Chédiak-Higashi syndrome	bacterial and fungal infections of skin and mucous membranes due to impaired leukocyte function

Albinism: Melanocytes are present but contain only unpigmented melanosomes.

1.13.) <u>AUTOSOMAL DOMINANT DISEASES</u>

familial hypercholesterolemia	abnormal LDL receptor ischemic heart disease
familial polyposis	colon cancer
spherocytosis	hemolytic anemia
von Willebrand disease	bleeding
Ehlers-Danlos syndrome	stretchy skin sprains, joint dislocations
Marfan syndrome	long bones lens dislocation
achondroplasia	premature ossification dwarfism: short limbs, normal trunk
phacomatoses	benign tumors of eye, skin and brain
Huntington's disease	chorea dementia
polycystic renal disease (adult type)	kidney failure

 Berry aneurysms are a/w <u>adult</u> type polycystic renal disease.

13

1.14.) X-LINKED RECESSIVE DISEASES

hemophilia A and B	bleeding
glucose-6-phosphate deficiency	hemolytic anemia
fragile X	mental retardation
Fabry disease	*sphingolipidosis* cardiomegaly angiokeratoma
Lesch-Nyhan syndrome	self mutilation gout
Duchenne, Becker	muscle dystrophy
Bruton's agammaglobulinemia	low or absent B cells
Wiskott-Aldrich syndrome	functional deficiency of B and T cells thrombocytopenia
chronic granulomatous disease	defect in neutrophil free radical formation

Fragile X chromosome: Small knob connected by a stalk to the main part of the chromosome which breaks off easily during karyotyping.
- Female carriers of fragile X may have slight mental retardation.
- Some affected males are mentally normal.

Female carriers of X-linked disorders are rarely affected because of the random inactivation of one of the X chromosomes in each cell (Lyon hypothesis).

1.15.) DELETIONS

Deletion of an entire autosomal chromosome is not compatible with life.

PARTIAL DELETIONS:

5p	cri du chat syndrome (newborn infants cry like kittens)
11p	congenital absence of iris
13q	retinoblastoma

p: short arm of chromosome
q: long arm of chromosome

A CURIOUS CASE:

Prader Willi syndrome	**15q11-13 deletion** **(paternal chromosome)** - severe infantile hypotony - obesity - mental retardation
Angelman syndrome	**15q11-13 deletion** **(maternal chromosome)** - "happy puppet" syndrome - happy smile, wide-based gait - epilepsy

It's a mystery! Why does a deletion of the maternally versus paternally derived chromosome 15 cause such a different phenotype?

1.16.) <u>HLA</u>

A3	hemochromatosis
B27	ankylosing spondylitis Reiter's syndrome ulcerative colitis
DR2	multiple sclerosis narcolepsy
DR3	SLE IDDM
DR4, Dw4, Dw14	rheumatoid arthritis juvenile rheumatoid arthritis

1.17.) <u>MOST COMMON CAUSES</u>

<u>MALIGNANCIES</u>:

	INCIDENCE	MORTALITY
men	prostate > lung > colon	lung > prostate > colon
women	breast > lung > colon	lung > breast > colon

 Skin cancers are the most common malignancies, but usually ignored from these statistics because of their low mortality.

<u>**Malignancies in children:**</u>
Most common malignancy **overall**:   leukemia (ALL)
Most common **solid** malignancy: brain tumors
Most common solid malignancy **outside CNS**:   neuroblastoma

<u>OTHER DISEASES</u>:

acute renal failure	tubular necrosis
nephrotic syndrome	**children** : minimal change glomerulonephritis **adults** : membranous glomerulonephritis
nephritic syndrome	poststreptococcal glomerulonephritis
hypertension	"idiopathic" > renal
anemia	iron deficiency
amenorrhea	pregnancy
chronic pancreatitis	alcoholism
food poisoning	*Clostridia perfringens* *Staph. aureus* toxin

Part B : Organ Pathology

1.18.) SLE

ANA	:	sensitive but not specific
anti ds-DNA and anti Sm	:	specific but not sensitive

CLINICAL FEATURES OF SLE:

1. Malar rash - spares nasolabial folds
2. Photosensitivity
3. Arthritis
   Pleuritis
   Pericarditis
4. Renal disease - proteinuria
5. Hemolytic anemia
   Leukopenia
   Lymphocytopenia
6. Antinuclear antibodies
7. False positive VDRL (cardiolipin antibodies)
   confirmed by negative FTA-ABS

LE cell:
Artificially injured leukocytes are mixed with patient's macrophages. Macrophages then phagocytose nuclei of injured leukocytes if the patient has SLE.

1.19.) SYSTEMIC SCLEROSIS

excessive fibrosis throughout the body

features	antibodies
a) limited = CREST localized scleroderma (fingers, forearm, face)	**anti-centromere**
b) diffuse systemic widespread scleroderma rapid progression early visceral involvement	**anti-Scl 70** (topoisomerase I)

 CREST: *Calcinosis*
Raynaud's
Esophageal dysmotility
Sclerodactyly
Telangiectasis

1.20.) SJÖGREN'S SYNDROME

immunological destruction of salivary and lacrimal glands

features	antibodies
dry eyes, dry mouth	**SS-A** (anti Ro) **SS-B** (anti La)

1.21.) <u>IMMUNODEFICIENCIES</u>

severe combined	lymphopenia (B and T)	X-linked or autosomal	death within first year
DiGeorge's	T cells absent	sporadic	viral infections fungal infections tetany
Bruton's	B cells absent	X-linked	bacterial infections
common variable	B cells present but produce few antibodies	variable	bacterial infections
IgA deficiency	low IgA	autosomal	sinopulmonary infections gastrointestinal infections
Wiskott-Aldrich	low IgM	X-recessive	bacterial infections thrombocytopenia eczema

- most common congenital immunodeficiency : IgA deficiency
- most common acquired immunodeficiency : AIDS

1.22.) <u>BLEEDING DISORDERS</u>

	key features
ITP (idiopathic thrombocytic purpura)	- immune mediated - children: acute (post viral infection) - adults: often chronic
TTP (thrombotic thrombocytic purpura)	- young women - microthrombi - fragmented RBCs (helmet cells)
lack of factor VIII-R (Von Willebrand disease)	**- aPTT prolonged** **- bleeding time prolonged**
lack of factor VIII (hemophilia A)	**- aPTT prolonged** - normal bleeding time
lack of factor IX (hemophilia B)	**- aPTT prolonged** - normal bleeding time
Vit. K deficiency (affects factors II, V, VII, IX, X)	**- PT prolonged** - fat malabsorption - antibiotics (diminished gut flora) - coumarin therapy

Bleeding Time:	platelet function
PT:	extrinsic + common pathways
aPTT:	intrinsic + common pathways
TT:	common pathway

1.23.) HEMOLYTIC ANEMIAS

A) HEREDITARY:

	key features
spherocytosis	- autosomal dominant - defective spectrin - splenomegaly

G6PD deficiency	- hemolysis during oxidative stress such as:
	   viral infections, fava beans,
	   sulfa drugs, quinine, nitrofurantoin
	- Heinz bodies (=hemoglobin degradation products)

sickle cell anemia	- **HbS** $(\alpha_2\beta^s_2)$ - sickling triggered by: hypoxia, dehydration, acidosis - vaso-occlusive crisis - aplastic crisis - sequestration crisis (splenomegaly) - autosplenectomy
α-Thalassemias	- **HbH** (β_4) - Hb Bart (γ_4), hydrops fetalis - common in Southeast Asia - hypochromic cells, target cells
β-Thalassemias[1]	- **HbA₂** $(\alpha_2\delta_2)$ and **HbF** $(\alpha_2\gamma_2)$ - common in Mediterranean and US - hypochromic cells, target cells

[1] **major** = homozygote, **minor** = heterozygote

B) IMMUNE MEDIATED:

warm antibodies (usually IgG)	cold antibodies (usually IgM)
active at 37°C	most active at 0~4°C
- drugs - malignancies - SLE	- mycoplasma pneumonia - mononucleosis - lymphoma

Cold antibodies: Agglutination occurs only in peripheral cool parts of the body -> vascular obstruction -> Raynaud's phenomenon.

COOMBS TEST:
direct test: detects cell bound antibodies
indirect test: detects free antibodies

1.24.) OTHER ANEMIAS

	key features
megaloblastic	- hypochromic, macrocytic RBCs - hypersegmented neutrophils - **folate** : anemia, no neurological symptoms - **B12** : anemia plus neurological symptoms
iron deficiency	- hypochromic, microcytic RBCs - chronic blood loss
aplastic (bone marrow failure)	- viral infections - toxins - drugs : alkylating agents chloramphenicol

 In elderly patients with iron deficiency anemia you should always suspect a colorectal malignancy!

Plummer-Vinson: anemia
+ atrophic glossitis
+ esophageal webs

Fanconi anemia: - autosomal recessive
- hypoplastic thumbs
- absent radii
- marrow DNA is more susceptible to radiation and alkylating agents -> patients develop aplastic anemia

1.25.) RED BLOOD CELLS

Heinz bodies (denatured hemoglobin)	- G6PD deficiency
Howell-Jolly bodies (nuclear fragments)	- post splenectomy
basophil stippling	- lead poisoning
siderocytes	- iron overload - Pappenheimer bodies
reticulocytes (remains of ribosomal RNA)	- increased production/release of RBCs - recovery from hemorrhage

Reticulocyte Index:
Following acute blood loss, the reticulocyte count may double within first 24h. It is important to relate the reticulocyte count to hematocrit in order to correct for the blood loss (so called "reticulocyte index").

1.26.) NEUTROPENIA

decreased production	- megaloblastic anemia - some leukemias, lymphomas
increased destruction	- immune mediated (Felty's syndrome)
drug induced	- alkylating agents - chloramphenicol - chlorpromazine - sulfonamides - phenylbutazone

1.27.) LEUKOCYTOSIS

neutrophils	- acute infections - stress
eosinophils	- allergy, asthma - parasitic infections
lymphocytes	- tuberculosis - viral infections
monocytes	- tuberculosis - malaria - rickettsia

1.28.) <u>LEUKEMIAS</u>

	ALL	AML	CML	CLL	hairy cell leukemia
	fever petechiae ecchymoses CNS infiltrate	fever petechiae ecchymoses lymphadenopathy (splenomegaly)	fever night sweats <u>splenomegaly</u>	insidious few symptoms low Ig levels infections	hepatomegaly splenomegaly
prognosis : fair		**poor**	**poor**	**fair**	**poor**
	lymphoblasts	Auer rods in myeloblasts	Philadelphia chro.	lymphocytes predominate	pancytopenia TRAP

<u>**Philadelphia chromosome:**</u>
c-abl protooncogene on chromosome 9 when translocated to the
breakpoint region (bcr) of chromosome 22 forms a fusion gene (bcr/abl).
This gene encodes a protein with high tyrosine kinase activity.

1.29.) LYMPHOMAS

Hodgkin's disease	Non-Hodgkin lymphoma
- spreads in contiguity - no leukemic component - Reed-Sternberg cells	- does not spread in contiguity - often has leukemic component

Reed-Sternberg cells*: Nobody knows where these cells come from!*
They are binucleated, have prominent nucleoli and clear parachromatin.

SUBTYPES HODGKIN:

	key features
a) lymphocyte predominance b) nodular sclerosis	these have better prognosis
c) mixed cellularity d) lymphocyte depletion	many Reed Sternberg cells -> poor prognosis

SUBTYPES NON-HODGKIN:

"many subtypes, several classifications, lots of confusion"

CLASS	EXAMPLE
low grade (good prognosis)	small lymphocytic lymphoma
intermediate grade	large cell lymphoma
high grade (poor prognosis)	immunoblastic lymphoma Burkitt lymphoma

---

"Starry sky" pattern of Burkitt lymphoma:
the "stars": benign macrophages
the "sky" : matrix of rapidly proliferating neoplastic B cells

---

1.30.) PLASMA CELL NEOPLASIAS

monoclonal gammopathy	multiple myeloma	Waldenström's
benign	malignant	malignant
usually IgG or IgA (may be IgM)	usually IgG or IgA (rarely IgD or IgE)	always IgM
<10% plasma cells in bone marrow	"myeloma cells" (>10% plasma cells infiltrating bone)	"flame cells" (eosinophilic plasma cells)
may convert to multiple myeloma	osteoclast activating factor (-> "punched-out" skull, pelvis, etc.)	hyperviscosity syndrome
	Bence-Jones proteins amyloidosis (tissue deposit of λ-chains)	

M-protein:
Monoclonal immunoglobulin secreted by single clone of aberrant plasma cells.
May be IgG, IgM etc.
Bence-Jones protein:
Excess light chains (unbalanced synthesis of immunoglobulins)
These are readily filtered through the glomeruli and appear in urine.

1.31.) PHLEBOTHROMBOSIS

Virchow's triad: - endothelial injury
- slow blood flow
- hypercoagulability

Trousseau's sign: - migratory venous thrombosis
- a/w neoplasms

1.32.) ARTERIOSCLEROSIS

	key features
atherosclerosis	- large and medium size arteries - fatty streaks - atheromas
Mönckeberg's	- media calcific stenosis - "gooseneck lumps" - small and medium size arteries - asymptomatic
arteriolosclerosis (hyperplastic)	- fibrinoid necrosis - malignant hypertension - "onion skin" hyperplasia
arteriolosclerosis (hyaline)	- diabetes, hypertension, old age - thickened basement membrane

1.33.) ARTERITIS

	key features
hypersensitivity arteritis	- small vessels - lesions all at same stage - cryoglobulins - a/w Henoch-Schönlein purpura
polyarteritis nodosa	- small and medium vessels - kidneys, heart, muscles, skin - can be fatal but responds well to steroids
thromboangiitis obliterans (Buerger's)	- small and medium vessels - in smokers
giant cell arteritis	**- temporal artery** - sudden blindness - female > male - a/w polymyalgia rheumatica
Wegener's	- upper respiratory vasculitis - lower respiratory vasculitis - glomerulonephritis
Takayasu	**- "pulseless disease"** - aorta / large arteries - Asian females
Kawasaki	**- mucocutaneous lymph node syndrome** - coronary artery aneurysms - fever, conjunctivitis, maculopapular rash - Japanese children

 Giant cell arteritis: *Early diagnosis is essential to prevent permanent loss of vision!*

1.34.) ANEURYSMS

	key features
atherosclerotic	- fusiform - abdominal aorta - hypertension
syphilitic	- saccular - ascending aorta - a/w aortic insufficiency
dissecting	- aorta (ascending or descending) - hypertension - Marfan syndrome
berry	- congenital - circle of Willis - a/w polycystic kidney disease (adult form)
micro	- cerebral : hypertension - retinal : diabetes

1.35.) <u>HEART SOUNDS</u>

	occurs in	sounds like
mitral valve prolapse	young women Marfan syndrome	midsystolic click
mitral stenosis	rheumatic heart disease atrial fibrillation	diastolic rumble
mitral regurgitation	MI (papillary muscle) acute rheumatic fever endocarditis	holosystolic murmur *transmitted to axilla*
aortic stenosis	congenital degenerative calcification	systolic murmur *transmitted to carotid art.*
aortic regurgitation	"water hammer" pulse	diastolic murmur "pistol shots" in femoral art.
patent ductus arteriosus	kept open by PGE_2 , PGI_2	continuous murmur (machine like)

 Pulsus parvus et tardus: *"small and weak" -> aortic stenosis*

1.36.) CONGENITAL HEART DEFECTS

A) TYPES

acyanotic (L -> R)	cyanotic (R -> L)	obstructive

- VSD [1]
 - ASD
   ostium primum
   ostium secundum
 	
 - PDA
	- Fallot's tetralogy [1]
	 - transposition of great vessels
	 - persistent truncus arteriosus
	 - Eisenmenger : reversal of
	   L->R shunt due to pulmonary
	   hypertension
		- coarctation of aorta
		   infants: preductal
		   adults: postductal
		
		 - pulmonary or aortic
		   stenosis or atresia

[1] most common cyanotic and acyanotic defects respectively

B) SYNDROMES A/W HEART DEFECTS

	cardiac defect plus
fetal alcohol syndrome	- microcephaly - short, upturned nose, long philtrum
fetal hydantoin syndrome	- microcephaly - nail hypoplasia
isotretinoin (Vit. A)	- hydrocephalus - cleft palate
TORCH (intrauterine infection)	- microcephaly - auditory and visual defects
syphilis	- bullous skin lesions (palms, soles) - Hutchinson's teeth - saber shins

> **TORCH:** Toxoplasmosis, Rubella, CMV, Herpes

1.37.) <u>ISCHEMIC HEART DISEASE</u>

	signs & treatment
stable angina	- exercise - ST depression - relieved by rest - *TX : nitroglycerin*
unstable angina	- at rest or crescendo like - often leads to MI - *unresponsive to nitroglycerin*
Prinzmetal's angina	- at rest - ST elevated - *TX : Ca^{2+} antagonists*

myocardial infarction	- during exercise or REM sleep
	- ST elevation
	- T inversion
	
	- *TX : nitroglycerin*
	     morphine
	     lidocaine

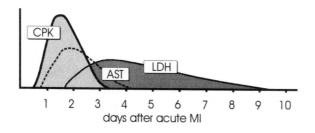

days after acute MI

1.38.) MYOCARDIAL INFARCTION

time after MI	gross change	microscopic change
30 minutes	-	mitochondrial swelling
4-12 h	-	edema, hemorrhage
18-24 h	pallor	neutrophilic infiltrate
24-72 h	pallor	coagulation necrosis loss of nuclei heavy neutrophil. Infiltrate
3-7 days	central softening hyperemic borders	resorption of dead myofibers
10 days	max. soft and yellow hyperemic borders	granulation tissue
8 weeks	gray and firm scar	scar

COMPLICATIONS:

Arrhythmia: most common cause of death in first hours after MI
Myocardial rupture: highest risk 1~2 weeks after MI

most common   *arrhythmia*
                   left heart failure
                   cardiogenic shock
least common   *muscle rupture*

36

1.39.) <u>HEART FAILURE</u>

LEFT	RIGHT
CAUSES:	
• ischemic heart disease • arterial hypertension • valvular disease	• left sided heart failure • lung disease • primary pulmonary hypertension
CONSEQUENCES:	
pulmonary congestion - dyspnea, orthopnea renal hypoperfusion - salt retention	increased venous pressure - edema - liver congestion ("nutmeg liver") -> ascites

1.40.) ENDOCARDITIS

acute	subacute	marantic	Libman Sacks
- *Staph. aureus* - *Streptococci*	- *Strep. viridans* - *gram negative bacilli*	- a/w chronic illnesses	- **SLE**
- previously normal valves	- previously abnormal valves	- thrombotic	- verrucous lesions on both sides of valve leaflets
- Janeway lesions	- Roth spots - Osler nodes		
- high fever, chills - hematuria	- low grade fever		

Janeway lesions: non-tender, macular patches on palms and soles (septic emboli)
Roth spots: oval retinal hemorrhages with pale center.
Osler nodes: red, tender lesions on finger and toe pulps.

1.41.) PERICARDITIS

	key features
fibrinous	- transmural myocardial infarction, - Dressler syndrome - "bread and butter" appearance
serous	- viral infections (coxsackie) - uremia
suppurative	- bacterial infections - fungal infections - parasitic infections

CLINICAL SIGNS:
- **pericardial friction rub**
- **pulsus paradoxus** (nothing paradox about it):
  a normal inspiratory fall in blood pressure that is <u>exaggerated</u>

Dressler syndrome: *Delayed pericarditis (2-10 weeks after infarction)*
due to auto-antibodies. Responds well to corticosteroids.

1.42.) <u>RHEUMATIC HEART DISEASE</u>

acute rheumatic fever	rheumatic heart disease
occurs 1-4 weeks after tonsillitis group A β-hemolytic streptococci	occurs many years after rheumatic fever often asymptomatic
common in children 5-15 years	fibrotic, deformed, calcified lines of closure on valve leaflets
major Jones criteria • **polyarthritis** • **erythema** • **subcutaneous nodules** • **chorea** • **carditis**	**mitral valve** > aortic valve

 <u>Carditis of rheumatic fever</u>:
pericarditis -> serous effusions
myocarditis -> heart failure
endocarditis -> valvular damage

<u>ASCHOFF BODY</u>:
- focal interstitial myocardial inflammation
- large myocytes (Anitschkow cells)
- multinucleated giant cells (Aschoff cells)

1.43.) <u>OBSTRUCTIVE LUNG DISEASES</u>

	key features
emphysema	- pink puffers , barrel chest - **panacinar** (α1-antitrypsin deficiency, lower lobes) - **centrilobular** (smoking, upper lobes)
chronic bronchitis	- blue bloaters - chronic irritation/ infections - hypertrophy of submucosal glands
asthma	- expiratory wheezing - extrinsic (triggered by allergens) - intrinsic (triggered by cold, exercise) [1] - aspirin induced
bronchiectasis	- result of chronic infections - Kartagener's : immotile cilia

[1] *intrinsic asthma is a common problem of ice skaters.*

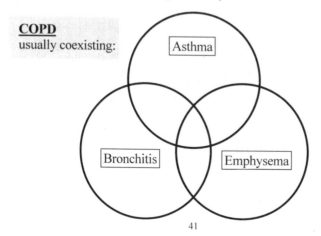

COPD
usually coexisting:

41

1.44.) RESTRICTIVE LUNG DISEASES

	key features
adult ARDS	- acute diffuse alveolar damage (causes: sepsis, shock, pancreatitis, toxins)
neonatal ARDS	- insufficient lecithin synthesis by type II pneumocytes
pneumoconiosis	- coal : "tattooing", black sputum - anthracosis : carbon dust - asbestosis : fibrous silicates, dry cough - berylliosis : **Type IV hypersensitivity**
hypersensitivity pneumonitis	- acute : **(Type III)** fever, cough, dyspnea, leukocytosis - chronic : **(Type IV)** peribronchial granulomas - farmer's lung, pigeon breeder's lung etc.
Goodpasture syndrome	- **(Type II)**, antibodies against basal membrane - hemoptysis, rapidly progressive glomerulonephritis
pulmonary hemosiderosis	- like Goodpasture's but without renal involvement
alveolar proteinosis	- overproduction of surfactant like material
eosinophilic pneumonia	- acute (Löffler's) : **Type 1 hypersensitivity** - chronic
diffuse idiopathic fibrosis	- interstitial pneumonitis and fibrosis - hyperplasia of type II pneumocytes
collagen vascular disorders	- scleroderma, SLE, Wegener's, RA etc.

1.45.) PNEUMONIA

	caused by
bronchopneumonia	*Hemophilus* *Pseudomonas*
lobar pneumonia	*Pneumococcus* *Klebsiella*
atypical pneumonia [1]	viral *Mycoplasma*
Legionnaire's disease [2] (self-limited lobar pneumonia)	*Legionella*

[1] most frequent in young adults (college students)

[2] more frequent in elderly, via water reservoirs
no person to person transmission

What is atypical about "atypical pneumonia"?
- more gradual onset
- dry, non productive cough
- minimal signs of pulmonary involvement during physical examination
- prominent extrapulmonary symptoms, myalgia etc.
- prominent chest x-ray ("looks worse than patient")

1.46.) LUNG TUMORS

benign	- hamartoma - adenoma - leiomyoma etc.
carcinoid	- potentially malignant - not related to smoking - <u>carcinoid syndrome</u> suggests widespread metastasis
carcinoma	**adeno CA** - peripheral, less related to smoking **squamous CA** - central, strong correlation with smoking **small cell CA** - central, hormone producing, aggressive **large cell CA** - peripheral, poorly differentiated adeno or squamous CA

<u>**Clinical features:**</u>
- less than 5% 10 year survival
- Pancoast tumor (apex of lung -> compressing cervical sympathetic chain -> Horner's syndrome)
- compression of recurrent laryngeal nerve -> hoarseness
- obstruction of superior vena cava -> facial swelling

PARANEOPLASTIC SYNDROMES:
small cell CA: ACTH
ADH
squamous CA: PTH-like factor

1.47.) <u>GLOMERULONEPHRITIS I</u>

nephritic syndrome	nephrotic syndrome
- hematuria - RBC casts	- severe proteinuria - hypoalbuminemia - hyperlipidemia - edema
- post streptococcal GN	- adults: membranous GN - children: minimal change GN

diffuse proliferative GN	- poststreptococcal GN - good prognosis
mesangiocapillary GN (membranoproliferative GN)	- young adults, idiopathic - poor prognosis
focal-segmental GN	- aggressive variant of minimal change GN
Goodpasture's (anti-GBM antibodies)	- young males - pulmonary hemorrhage
Berger's (IgA nephropathy)	- extremely common, lasts 1-2 days - mild proteinuria, hematuria in children - follows respiratory infection

1.48.) GLOMERULONEPHRITIS II

	clinical features	pathologic features	prognosis
minimal change (lipoid nephrosis)	- most common nephrotic syndrome in children - insidious onset	- no immune complexes - **loss of foot processes**	good
membranous	- most common nephrotic syndrome in young adults - insidious onset	- thickening of GBM - **subepithelial** deposits of immune complexes - 85% unknown antigen	mixed
membranoproliferative	- variable presentation	- GBM thickening plus proliferation of mesangium - **subendothelial or intra-membranous** deposits of immune complexes - "tram track" appearance	very poor
focal segmental	- maybe related to minimal change - but proteinuria is nonselective	- segmental sclerosis - usually IgM deposits (**IgA in Berger's**)	poor
diffuse proliferative	- nephritic/nephrotic - post streptococcal, SLE	- proliferation of mesangium and epithelium - **subepithelial** deposits	good
rapidly progressive	- aggressive variant of other GN	- **crescents** - oliguria, uremia	very poor

1.49.) <u>UROLITHIASIS</u>

calcium	- 80% of cases - precipitates in **alkaline** urine - *TX : thiazide* *potassium phosphate*

Mg - NH$_3$ - Phosphate	- "triple stones"
	  (staghorn calculi)
	- urinary tract infections (*Proteus*)
	- precipitates in **alkaline** urine
	
	- *TX : antibiotics*
	  acidification

uric acid	- gout - leukemia - precipitates in **acidic** urine - *TX : bicarbonate*
cystine	- congenital defect in dibasic amino acid transporter - precipitates in **acidic** urine - *TX : bicarbonate*

1.50.) VENEREAL DISEASES

	caused by	clinical features	treatment
condyloma acuminatum	HPV	"red warts"	cryotherapy
syphilis (I) **syphilis (II)** **syphilis (III)**	*Treponema pallidum*	hard chancre (**painless**) cond. lata (flat brown papules) gumma	penicillin G
chancroid	*Hemophilus ducreyi*	soft chancre (**painful**)	ceftriaxone
lymphogranuloma venereum	*Chlamydia trachomatis*	ulcer (**painless**) lymphadenopathy	doxycycline
granuloma inguinale	*C. donovani*	multiple ulcerating papules lymph nodes not involved [1]	tetracycline
trichomoniasis	*Trichomonas vaginalis*	men : asymptomatic or NGU female : vaginitis	metronidazole
genital herpes	HSV2 or HSV1	recurrent vesicles (**painful**)	acyclovir
candidiasis [2]	*Candida albicans*	female : vaginitis	miconazole, nystatin

[1] induration is of subcutaneous tissue   [2] listed for comparison only - candidiasis is not sexually transmitted

48

1.51.) <u>TESTES TUMORS</u>

GERM CELL TUMORS (common)

	key features
seminoma	- uniform polyhedral - radiosensitive, often curable
embryonal	- more aggressive - hemorrhage, necrosis
choriocarcinoma	- highly malignant - gynecomastia
yolk sac	- most common in children - serum AFP ↑ - very aggressive
teratoma	- contains multiple tissue types - often malignant!

NON GERM CELL TUMORS (rare)

Leydig cell	- androgens, estrogens, corticosteroids - usually benign
Sertoli cell	- little or no hormone production
lymphoma	- most common in elderly

> **<u>Tumor markers:</u>**
> **AFP:** all germ cell CA except choriocarcinoma
> **HCG:** all germ cell CA except yolk sac carcinoma

1.52.) <u>OVARIAN TUMORS</u>

SURFACE ENDOTHELIUM (most common)

	key features
serous	- cysts, ciliated epithelium
mucinous	- cysts, non ciliated epithelium
endometrioid	- glandular tissue
clear cell	- rare, malignant
Brenner	- rare, benign - nests of <u>transitional</u> epithelium in stroma

GERM CELL TUMORS (less common)

teratoma	- usually mature (benign) [1]
dysgerminoma	= seminoma, radiosensitive
endodermal sinus tumor	= yolk sac tumor, AFP ↑
choriocarcinoma	HCG

[1] also called dermoid cyst

SEX CORD STROMA CELL TUMORS (rare)

granulosa-theca	estrogens and androgens
Sertoli-Leydig	androgens -> masculinization
fibroma	Meig's syndrome -> ascites

1.53.) ENDOMETRIUM

polyps	hyperplasia	carcinoma
- excessive bleeding - rarely malignant transformation	- excessive bleeding - premalignant	- usually adenocarcinoma - may be asymptomatic or or present with bleeding
		risk factors age >40 years early menarche late menopause nulliparity obesity

1.54.) PLACENTA

hydatidiform mole	choriocarcinoma
- older pregnant woman - uterus larger than expected - grape-like cystic material - 80% benign	- derived from : hydatidiform mole (50%) pregnancy (25%) abortion (25%)
- HCG elevated	- HCG elevated - frequent metastases

complete hydatidiform mole:
karyotype 46,XX of exclusively paternal origin

incomplete hydatidiform mole:
embryo present (triploid or tetraploid cells)
due to fertilization of ovum by multiple sperm cells

1.55.) BREAST

fibrocystic change	breast cancer
- often bilateral - multiple nodules - menstrual variation - may regress during pregnancy	- often unilateral - single mass - no cyclic variations

BENIGN TUMORS

fibroadenoma	- single, movable nodule
cystosarcoma phyllodes	- rapidly growing, may become huge
intraductal papilloma	- nipple discharge (bloody or serous) - nipple retraction

MALIGNANT TUMORS

ductal carcinoma	- most common
lobular carcinoma	- often receptor positive
Paget's	- older woman - nipple involved - poor prognosis

Risk factors for breast cancer
- positive family history
- early menarche
- late menopause
- nulliparity
- (high animal fat diet)

1.56.) <u>MOUTH</u>

bleeding gums	Vit. C deficiency
glossitis, cheilosis	Vit. B2 deficiency
smooth beefy red tongue	Vit. B12 deficiency
strawberry tongue	scarlet fever
Koplik's spots (white dots on red background)	measles
thrush (white, removable)	Candida albicans

1.57.) <u>ESOPHAGEAL DIVERTICULA</u>

Pulsion Diverticula (Zenker's)	Traction Diverticula
- "false" (mucosa only)	- "true" (all layers)
- at junction of pharynx/esophagus	- mid part of esophagus
- dysphagia, regurgitation	- asymptomatic

1.58.) <u>GASTRITIS</u>

acute erosive	chronic type A	chronic type B	Ménétrier's
- focal damage - alcohol - NSAIDs - stress	- fundal gastritis - autoimmune - pernicious anemia - achlorhydria	- antral gastritis - *H. pylori*	- thickened mucosa

 Patients on intensive care often develop acute erosive gastritis.

> **_H. pylori_ is associated with:**
> - chronic gastritis type B
> - gastric and duodenal peptic ulcers
> - carcinoma of stomach

1.59.) <u>GASTROENTERITIS</u>

toxin ingestion	bacteria	non-bacterial
Staph. aureus *Cl. botulinum*	toxigenic *Campylobacter* *E. coli* *Salmonella* invasive *Shigella*	Rotavirus (children) Parvovirus (adults) *Candida* *Entameba histolytica* *Giardia lamblia*

55

1.60.) POLYPOSIS OF COLON

		polyps plus:	cancer risk:
familial multiple polyposis	autosomal dominant	- (none)	almost 100%
Gardner's	autosomal dominant	- skin and bone tumors	almost 100%
Turcot's	autosomal recessive	- brain tumors	high
Peutz-Jeghers	autosomal dominant	- melanin pigmentation of lips, palms and soles	very low

Familial polyposis:
- Patient's off-spring has 50% risk of disease:
- Screen annually until age 35 (flexible sigmoidoscopy).
- If polyps develop -> need to remove colon.

1.61.) <u>INFLAMMATORY BOWEL DISEASE</u>

CROHN'S DISEASE	ULCERATIVE COLITIS
rectum often spared **ileum often involved**	**begins at rectum and progresses** **towards ileocecal junction**
skip lesions transmural	continuous mucosa / submucosa only
granulomas strictures and fissures	crypt abscesses pseudopolyps
more **pain**, less bleeding	more **bleeding**, less pain
	complications: - increased risk of colon carcinoma - toxic megacolon

Common extraintestinal manifestations of CD and UC:
- arthritis, iritis, sclerosing cholangitis

1.62.) <u>MALABSORPTION</u>

celiac sprue	- toxic/allergic reaction against gluten - flat mucosal surface - avoid wheat - rice and corn are o.k.
tropical sprue	- *E. coli* enterotoxin ?
Whipple's disease	- systemic disease - arthritis is common - PAS positive macrophages in mucosa - *TX : penicillin or tetracycline*

1.63.) <u>CHOLELITHIASIS</u>

STONE TYPES:

cholesterol	mixed	pigment (bilirubin)
- radiolucent [1] - often a single stone - Westerners - **fat, female, forty, fertile**	- most common - 15% radiopaque	- radiolucent [1] - a/w hemolytic anemia - Asians

[1] not detectable on plain radiograph

Porcelain Gallbladder: - calcium deposits in wall
- high risk of malignancy

Strawberry Gallbladder: - asymptomatic lipid deposits
- not related to cholelithiasis
- no cancer risk

Charcot's triad (cholangitis):
- *acute onset fever, sepsis*
- *RUQ pain*
- *jaundice*

1.64.) <u>CARCINOMA</u>

gallbladder CA	bile duct CA
- female - cholelithiasis - porcelain gallbladder	- male - chronic infections - liver fluke (*Clonorchis sinensis*)

1.65.) JAUNDICE

occurs when serum bilirubin > 2 mg/dl
direct   = conjugated   = water soluble
indirect = unconjugated = insoluble (bound to albumin)

	due to	serum bilirubin
prehepatic	hemolysis	unconjugated
hepatic	hepatitis	conjugated and unconjugated
posthepatic	cholestasis	conjugated

Congenital causes of jaundice :

Gilbert	auto-dominant	impaired uptake (mild)
Crigler-Najjar	auto-dominant or auto-recessive	impaired uptake (very severe)
Rotor	auto-recessive	impaired hepatocellular secretion

Physiologic jaundice of the newborn:
- *onset 2-3 days after birth*
- *peak < 12 mg/dL*
- *persists < 1 week*
- *more severe in prematures*

1.66.) <u>HEPATITIS</u>

A	RNA	- viruses in feces - acute : IgM - late : IgG	- **fecal/oral** - 2-6 weeks [2] - 0% chronic
B	DNA	- HBs-Ag , earliest marker[1] - HBe-Ag, infective state	- **parenteral** - 2-6 months [2] - 10% chronic
C	RNA	- antibody ELISA	- **parenteral** - 1-2 months [2] - 50% chronic
Delta	RNA	- requires HBV's Ag coat (superinfection)	- **parenteral**
E	RNA		- **fecal oral** - SE Asia - often fulminant in pregnant woman

[1] also indicates carrier state   [2] incubation times

CHRONIC HEPATITIS (> 6 months):
chronic persistent hepatitis
- inflammation limited to portal triad

chronic active hepatitis
- inflammation beyond portal triad
  (piece meal necrosis)

1.67.) <u>HEPATITIS B SEROLOGY</u>

HBeAg	- appears after HBsAg - disappears before HBsAg - indicates infectivity!
HBsAg	- appears before onset of symptoms - persists for 3-4 months - if > 6 months: chronic carrier state
anti-HBsAg	- appears a few weeks after HBsAg has disappeared - indicates recovery and immunity
anti HBcAg	- only marker present during "window period"

*"**Window period**": time after HBsAg disappears but before anti-HBsAg appears in patient's serum.*

1.68.) <u>TOXIC HEPATITIS</u>

predictable	idiosyncratic
amanita acetaminophen carbon tetrachloride methotrexate	halothane isoniazid methyl-DOPA

1.69.) CIRRHOSIS

MOST COMMON TYPES OF CIRRHOSIS:

alcohol (60%)	toxins, viral (30%)	biliary (10%)
early : micronodular late : macronodular	macronodular	micronodular
Mallory bodies in acute hepatitis !		autoimmune disease anti-mitochondrial antibodies

RARE TYPES OF CIRRHOSIS:

Hemochromatosis: - accumulation of hemosiderin
- triad of cirrhosis, diabetes mellitus and skin pigmentation

Wilson's disease: - accumulation of copper
- decreased serum ceruloplasmin

1.70.) LIVER CARCINOMA

metastatic	hepatocellular	cholangiocarcinoma
most common	90% of all primary ones	10% of primary ones
from breast **from lung** **from colon**	HBV and HCV aflatoxin	more common in Asia (liver fluke)
	AFP ↑	

1.71.) <u>ARTHRITIS</u>

osteoarthritis	rheumatoid arthritis (RA)
- women > men	- women 20~50 years

- loss of cartilage
- narrowing of joint space
- increased density of subchondral bone
- osteophyte formation
	- synovial membrane proliferation
	  (pannus)
	- erosions of cartilage and
	  subchondral bone

- knees, hips, spine - distal interphalangeal joints	- starts in small joints - proximal interphalangeal joints - metacarpophalangeal joints
- joint stiffness after inactivity (e.g. sitting in chair) - Heberden's nodes	- morning stiffness - soft tissue swelling - rheumatoid nodules (skin, valves..) - **rheumatoid factor**: anti IgG

 Heberden's nodes are osteophytes at the distal interphalangeal joints.

> **Still's disease:**
> juvenile RA, acute febrile, no rheumatoid factors
>
> **Psoriatic arthritis:**
> like RA, but absence of rheumatoid factors
>
> **Felty's syndrome:**
> polyarticular RA, splenomegaly, leukopenia, leg ulcers

1.72.) <u>BONES</u>

	key features
osteogenesis imperfecta	- disorder of collagen synthesis - fractures - blue, thin sclera
osteopetrosis	- increased density - brittle bones
achondroplasia	- autosomal dominant - defective cartilage synthesis - decreased epiphyseal formation - short limbs, normal size head and trunk

aseptic necrosis	- secondary to trauma:
	  head of femur
	  navicular bone

osteoporosis	osteomalacia	Paget's
- thinned cortical bone - enlarged medullary cavity	- diffuse radiolucency	- bones enlarged and radiolucent
- normal Ca and phosphate - normal alk. phosphatase	- low Ca, low phosphate - high alk. phosphatase	- extremely high alkaline phosphatase

- decreased bone mass
- estrogen deficiency
- immobilization
- Cushing's syndrome
	- impaired mineralization
	- lack of Vit. D
	- chronic renal
	  insufficiency
		- excessive bone resorption
		  with replacement.

1.73.) CARTILAGE

TYPES OF CARTILAGE:

hyaline cartilage	most common type - *joints* - *developing bones* - *joints* - *trachea/larynx* - *nose*
fibrocartilage	contains type I collagen fibers - *intervertebral disks* - *menisci*
elastic cartilage	contains elastin - *ear*

TUMORS:

	key features
osteochondroma	- developmental defect - exostosis at metaphyseal projections
enchondroma	- may develop into chondrosarcoma - cartilage within bone
chondroblastoma	- benign - femur, tibia, humerus epiphysis
chondrosarcoma	- malignant - spine, pelvic bones - slower growing than osteosarcoma

1.74.) <u>BONE TUMORS</u>

	key features
osteoma	- benign - skull
osteoid osteoma	- benign, painful - tibia or femur (diaphysis)
osteoblastoma	- like osteoid osteoma - larger but painless - may be malignant
osteosarcoma	- highly malignant - metaphysis of long bone (knee) - Codman's triangle
Ewing's sarcoma	- very aggressive - young males - pelvis, long bones - within marrow cavity - "onion skin" appearance

1.75.) <u>MUSCULAR DYSTROPHIES</u>

	key features
Duchenne	**- X linked** **- abnormal dystrophin protein** - most severe - pelvic girdle weakness - pseudohypertrophy of calves
Becker	**- X linked** **- abnormal dystrophin protein** - less severe than Duchenne - may walk until age 20-25
limb girdle	**- autosomal recessive** - late onset
facioscapulohumeral	**- autosomal dominant** - late onset
myotonic	**- autosomal dominant** - late onset - limb involvement is distal - inability to voluntarily relax muscle

 Gower's sign*: When trying to stand up the child uses its hands to climb up himself.*

<u>CLINICAL FEATURES (Duchenne):</u>
- presents in boys age 3-7
- proximal muscle weakness -> waddling gait
- pseudohypertrophy: fatty and fibrous infiltration of calve muscle
- increased serum CPK

1.76.) BRAIN TUMORS

		key features
Neural Tube (gliomas)	astrocytoma	- slow growing, M > F
	glioblastoma	- always fatal, M > F
	medulloblastoma	- children, M > F
	oligodendroblastoma	- rare, M = F slow growing, seizures
Neural Crest	meningioma	- from arachnoid, benign, F > M "whorling pattern", psammoma bodies
	Schwannoma	- acoustic neurinoma, F > M a/w von Recklinghausen's
	neurofibroma	- fibroblasts and Schwann cells, benign usually von Recklinghausen's
Ectoderm	craniopharyngioma	- most common supratentorial tumor in children, compresses optic nerve
	pituitary adenoma	- 60% prolactin (chromophobe) - 10% growth hormone (eosinophil) - 10% ACTH (basophil)
Mesoderm	lymphoma	- B cells, periventricular
	lipoma	- "egg shell" appearance
	hemangioblastoma	

1.77.) <u>CNS DEGENERATION</u>

	key features
Alzheimer's	- most common - diffuse cortical atrophy
Pick's	- lobar atrophy - mainly frontal and temporal
Parkinson's	- bradykinesia, rigidity, resting tremor - dopamine depletion (caudate, putamen) - Lewy bodies
ALS	- rapidly progressive - degeneration of corticospinal tract (UMN) - degeneration of α-motoneurons (LMN)
Huntington's	- chorea, athetoid movements - atrophy of caudate, putamen and frontal cortex
Friedreich's ataxia	- autosomal recessive - pes cavus - loss of proprioception - tremors, Babinski reflex - spinal cord atrophy (spinocerebellar, corticospinal, post. columns)

- ***Upper motor neuron lesions:*** *spasticity, increased tendon reflexes*
- ***Lower motor neuron lesions:*** *paralysis, fasciculations, absent tendon reflexes*

1.78.) <u>DEMYELINATING DISEASES</u>

	key features
multiple sclerosis	- onset at age 20-40 - a/w cool, temperate climate - oligoclonal bands
Devic's	- like MS, but limited to spinal chord and optical nerve
Guillain-Barré	- peripheral nerves (mainly motor) - autoimmune, often following viral infection
adrenoleukodystrophy	- X linked - accumulation of long chain cholesterols - blindness, ataxia - latent adrenal insufficiency
Schilder's	- focal demyelination in brain - children - visual, auditory, motor defects - variant of adrenoleukodystrophy

---

<u>Oligoclonal bands (CSF electrophoresis)</u>:
- Multiple monoclonal gamma globulins.
- However, these are not entirely specific for MS.

1.79.) PITUITARY HYPERFUNCTION

eosinophile cells	prolactin	male : decreased libido, impotence female : galactorrhea, amenorrhea, infertility
	GH	prepubertal : giantism adults : acromegaly
basophile cells	ACTH	Cushing's disease: is the most common cause of Cushing's syndrome (except iatrogenic)

Classification according to staining properties is outdated since there is only an approximate relationship between hormones and cell staining.

While prolactin is mainly produced by eosinophil cells, prolactinomas are usually **chromophobe** *!*

1.80.) PITUITARY HYPOFUNCTION

Sheehan's syndrome (ischemic necrosis, postpartum)	panhypopituitarism - hypothyroidism - hypoadrenalism - hypogonadism
dwarfism	a) growth hormone deficiency b) lack of receptors (e.g. in pygmies)
eunuchoid hypogonadism, primary amenorrhea	gonadotropin deficiency (common !)

1.81.) ADRENAL ADENOMAS/CARCINOMAS

cortex : adenoma	most adenomas do not produce steroids - **Conn** : mineralocorticoids - **Cushing** : glucocorticoids - **virilization** : androgens
cortex : carcinoma	much rarer than adenomas, but if they occur they usually produce hormones!
medulla : pheochromocytoma	10% extra-adrenal 10% bilateral 10% malignant
medulla : neuroblastoma	malignant medulla or sympathetic chain ganglia

Conn: - hypernatremia -> hypervolemia -> high blood pressure
- potassium loss -> muscle weakness

Cushing: - "moon facies", "buffalo hump"
- truncal obesity
- skin striae
- osteoporosis
- low glucose tolerance

Mineral corticoids	zona **Glomerulosa**
Glucocorticoids	zona **Fasciculata**
Androgens	zona **Reticularis**

"the deeper you go the sweeter it gets"

1.82.) THYROID

		key features
hyperthyroidism :	**Graves'** (diffuse toxic goiter)	- lymphocytes - small follicles - little colloid
	Plummer's (nodular toxic goiter)	- hyperplasia, hypertrophy - colloid accumulation
hypothyroidism :	**diffuse simple goiter** (iodine deficiency)	- hyperplasia, hypertrophy
	Hashimoto's	- lymphocytes, plasma cells - atrophic follicles - little colloid
	Riedel's	- fibrous replacement
euthyroid :	**De Quervain's**	- viral - leakage of colloid - granulomas

"Sick euthyroid" syndrome:
- Many patients with severe illness, trauma or stress have low T3 and low T4, but clinically no signs of hypothyroidism.
- TSH is also normal in these cases.

1.83.) THYROID TUMORS

		key features
benign :	follicular adenoma	- very common - most are cold nodules
malignant :	papillary CA	- younger patients - a/w radiation exposure - Psammoma bodies
	follicular CA	- adenomatous pattern
	anaplastic CA	- undifferentiated - poor prognosis
	medullary CA	- parafollicular (C cells)

 Medullary CA of the thyroid is often a/w MEN type II.

- Papillary carcinoma is more common than follicular carcinoma.
- Follicular carcinoma is more aggressive than papillary carcinoma.

1.84.) <u>PARATHYROIDS</u>

	key features
hyperparathyroidism	**<u>primary</u>** - adenoma (usually) **<u>secondary</u>** - chronic renal failure - Vit. D deficiency
hypoparathyroidism	- thyroidectomy, radiation - DiGeorge's syndrome - **PTH low** - **Ca^{2+} low**
pseudohypo...	- receptor defect - short stature - short metacarpal bones - **PTH elevated** - **Ca^{2+} low**
pseudopseudohypo...	- same physical appearance as in pseudohypoparathyroidism - **PTH normal** - **Ca^{2+} levels normal**

<u>RENAL OSTEODYSTROPHY</u>:
chronic renal failure -> decreased phosphate excretion
                       -> phosphate binds ionized calcium in serum
                       -> hypocalcemia
                       -> increased PTH
                       -> bone demineralization

TX: Aluminum may be used to bind phosphate.

1.85.) <u>DIABETES MELLITUS</u>

A) PRIMARY:

IDDM (Type I)	NIDDM (Type II)	MODY
- not so common	- very common	- rare
- juvenile onset - prone to ketoacidosis	- adult onset - not prone to ketoacidosis	- juvenile onset
- viral etiology?	- inadequate insulin secretion - obesity, insulin resistance	- glucokinase defect (glucose sensor)
- strong genetic predisposition - auto-immune (islet cell antibodies)	- weak genetic predisposition (HLA DR 3, DR4)	
- decreased number of β-cells	- hyalinization of islets	

B) SECONDARY DIABETES:

hemochromatosis	chronic pancreatitis, pancreas carcinoma
"bronze diabetes"	-> islet cell destruction

Gestational diabetes: 1-3% of women develop diabetes during pregnancy. This induces excessive fetal insulin secretion and increases the risk of birth trauma (increased fetal weight due to the metabolic effects of insulin).
Usually glucose tolerance returns to normal after delivery, but 30% of women with gestational diabetes develop overt diabetes mellitus within 5 years.

1.86.) <u>MULTIPLE ENDOCRINE NEOPLASIA</u>
(autosomal dominant diseases)

MEN Type 1	MEN Type 2A	MEN Type 2B
adrenal <u>cortex</u> pituitary parathyroid pancreas (gastrinoma)	adrenal <u>medulla</u> thyroid medulla parathyroid	adrenal <u>medulla</u> thyroid medulla mucosal neuromas marfanoid features
"pity-para-pan"	"para-medullary-medulla"	

<u>CLINICAL PRESENTATIONS:</u>

MEN 1:   (90%) primary hyperparathyroidism -> hypercalcemia
(70%) gastrin -> Zollinger-Ellison syndrome -> peptic ulcers
(60%) pituitary tumors -> visual disturbances
         (sometimes produce GH -> acromegaly)

MEN 2A: (100%) medullary carcinoma of thyroid (bilateral)
            - early diagnosis is essential!
(50%)   benign pheochromocytoma (bilateral)
            -> hypertensive crisis (headache, sweating, palpitations)
(20%)   primary hyperparathyroidism -> hypercalcemia

Hypercalcemia is usually asymptomatic or may produce kidney stones.

1.87.) SKIN CANCER

	key features
seborrheic keratosis	- brownish/gray, scaly, greasy
keratoacanthoma	- rapidly growing pink papula - looks like squamous cell carcinoma but is benign
actinic keratosis	- crusty red papule, premalignant
basal cell carcinoma	- pearly, gray papule
squamous cell carcinoma	- erythematous, scaly or oozing ulcer - Bowen's disease: squamous CA in situ
melanoma	- brown, black, red, white, purple, irregular borders - lentigo maligna : grows horizontally - nodular melanoma : grows vertically

The "ABC" of melanoma:
A - asymmetric lesion
B - borders irregular
C - color variations

1.88.) OTHER SKIN DISEASES

	key features
pemphigus	- vesicles on mucosa - auto antibodies against intercellular junctions of keratinocytes
pemphigoid	- like pemphigus, but larger bullae on abdomen and groin
impetigo	- honey colored crust, superficial skin infection - *Staph.* or β-hemolytic *Strep.*
pityriasis	- (viral cause?) - herald patch -> spreads along flexural lines
rosacea	- large, red nose

	key features
xanthoma	- hyperlipidemia, foamy histocytes
capillary hemangioma	- "salmon patches" and stork bites *spontaneously regresses* - "strawberry hemangiomas" *initially grows, later regresses*
cavernous hemangioma	- "port-wine stain", a/w Sturge-Weber *does not resolve spontaneously*
cafe au lait spots	- a/w von Recklinghausen's
vitiligo	- irregular depigmentation

1.89.) <u>TOXINS</u>

cadmium	"honeycomb" pneumonitis
cobalt	cardiomyopathy
lead	inhibits heme synthesis renal tubular acidosis
mercury	neurotoxic (Minamata !) proximal tubular necrosis
arsenic	lung cancer
asbestos	mesothelioma
aromatic amines	bladder cancer
benzene	leukemia
chromium	lung cancer
vinyl chloride	liver angiosarcoma
CO	forms carboxyhemoglobin [1]
α-amanitin	fulminant hepatitis

[1] do not confuse with methemoglobin, which contains oxidized Fe^{3+}

Hot-Pics

> **Be able to recognize the following pictures:**

MICROSCOPIC:

- **Amyloid:** birefringence
- **Red blood cells:** microcytic hypochrome versus macrocytic megaloblastic
    target cells
    sickle cells
- **White blood cells:** ALL versus AML
- **Reed-Sternberg cell** (Hodgkin's disease)
- **Barrett's esophagus:** metaplasia
- **Granulomas:** caseating (TBC) versus non-caseating (foreign body)
- **Lung:** acid fast bacilli
    Aspergillus,
    Pneumocystis carinii (silver stain)
- **Lung:** oat cell carcinoma
- **Breast:** normal versus fibroadenoma versus cancer
- **Kaposi sarcoma**
- **Teratoma:** skin, teeth, neural tissue etc.
- **Giant cell arteritis**
- **Bacterial pneumonia**
- **Kidneys:** hypertensive change
- **Kidney immunofluorescence**: linear pattern (Goodpasture's syndrome)
    granular pattern (membranous GN)
    mesangial pattern (IgA nephropathy)
- **Colon:** adenomatous polyp versus adenocarcinoma
- **Liver:** hepatitis, fatty degeneration
- **Ovary:** Krukenberg tumor (signet ring cells)
- **Cervix:** carcinoma in situ
- **Pap smear:** dysplastic cell versus glycogen rich normal cells
- **CNS:** Alzheimer's disease: neurofibrillary tangles, plaques
    Parkinson's disease: depigmentation of substantia nigra

MACROSCOPIC:

- **Cardiac hypertrophy:** eccentric versus concentric hypertrophy
- **Breast carcinoma:** (mammography)
- **Lung:** Ghon complex (X-ray)
- **Gall-bladder:** stone types
- **Hydatidiform mole**
- **Pituitary adenoma** (X-ray of sella turcica)
- **Brain:** - atrophy of cortex
  - atrophy of caudate nucleus

MICROBIOLOGY

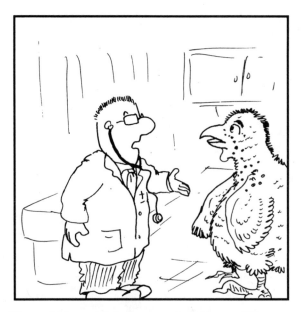

"It could be chicken pox, but then all these
viruses look similar."

Part A : General Microbiology

2.1.) STAINS

	used for
Ziehl Neelsen	stains acid fast bacteria red
India ink	cryptococcus
Giemsa	blood smears
PAS	glycogen, mucopolysaccharides
Prussian blue	iron
Congo red	amyloid
osmic acid	for electron microscopy

> **Gram stain:**
> 1. Crystal violet dye (plus iodine) stains all bacterial cell walls.
> 2. Alcohol extracts blue dye from lipid-rich, thin-walled gram-negative bacteria.
> 3. Red dye counterstains decolorized gram-negative bacteria. Gram-positive bacteria remain blue.

2.2.) <u>NORMAL FLORA</u>

Benefits of indigenous flora: *- stimulates immune system*
- interferes with pathogenic strains

	usual flora	potential pathogens
skin	Staph. epidermidis	Staph. aureus
nasopharynx	Strep. viridans anaerobes	Strep. pneumoniae N. meningitides H. influenzae
mouth	Strep. viridans	Candida albicans
colon	E. coli	Bacteroides fragilis enterococci
vagina	Lactobacillus Streptococci	Candida albicans

<u>Clinical examples:</u>
- Risk of endocarditis after dental procedures (*Strep. viridans*)
- Pseudomembranous colitis following administration of broad-spectrum antibiotics (*Cl. difficile* usually suppressed by endogenous flora)

2.3.) CELL WALLS

all bacteria (except mycoplasma)	**- inner layer of cell wall**: peptidoglycans (thick in gram-positives) (thin in gram-negatives)
gram positive	**- outer layer of cell wall**: teichoic acid
gram negative	**- outer layer of cell wall**: lipopolysaccharides (= endotoxins) - outer cell membrane (lipid bilayer) [1] - porins
mycobacteria	- mycolic acid in cell wall (resists decoloration of gram-stain)
mycoplasma	- have no cell wall - membrane contains sterols
spores	- dipicolinic acid (keratin coat) -> resistance to heat, dehydration and chemicals

[1] the space between outer membrane and cell membrane contains β-lactamase (degrades penicillins).

Cell capsule: composed of polysaccharides
- determines virulence
- capsular antigens determine species
- vaccines are made against capsular antigens

2.4.) <u>TOXINS</u>

ENDOTOXINS	- **lipopolysaccharides** - **non-specific** - TNF, IL-1 --> fever, shock - poor antigen - heat stabile
EXOTOXINS	- **polypeptides** - **specific** - toxoids used as vaccine - usually heat labile
tetanus toxin	- blocks release of glycine -> muscle spasms
botulinum toxin	- blocks release of ACh -> muscle paralysis
diphtheria toxin	- inhibits protein synthesis - (ADP-ribosylation of EF-2)
alpha toxin	- *Staph. aureus* - hemolysis, necrosis, cell death
toxic shock syndrome toxin	- *Staph. aureus* - induces cytokines -> shock
cholera toxin	- stimulates adenylate cyclase (activates G_s)
pertussis toxin	- stimulates adenylate cyclase (inhibits G_i)
enterotoxin	- *E. coli* - heat labile: stimulates adenylate cyclase - heat stable: stimulates guanylate cyclase

2.5.) O$_2$-REQUIREMENTS

obligate aerobe	M. tuberculosis B. anthracis Nocardia
micro aerophilic	Brucella abortus Campylobacter jejuni
obligate anaerobe	Clostridium Actinomyces
facultative anaerobe	most others

Reactivation of tuberculosis usually appears in the better ventilated upper lobes of the lung!

2.6) <u>MOST COMMON CAUSES</u>

common cold	rhino viruses
pharyngitis, laryngitis	viral > bacterial (ß-hemolyzing Strept.)
tonsillitis	ß-hemolyzing Strept.
sinusitis	Strep. pneumoniae, Staph. aureus
otitis media	Strep. pneumoniae, Hemophilus influenza
bronchitis	Hemophilus influenza, Strep. pneumoniae
pneumonia - infants **- young adults** **- elderly**	**- RSV** **- mycoplasma** **- Strep. pneumoniae**
meningitis - neonates **- infants** **- adults** **- elderly** **- overall**	**- Strep. agalactia, E. coli** **- Hemophilus influenza** **- Neisseria meningitidis** **- Strep. pneumoniae** **- Hemophilus influenza**
encephalitis	viral
endocarditis	Strep. viridans
post transfusion hepatitis	hepatitis C
carbuncle	Staph. aureus
sepsis (catheterized patient)	Staph. aureus, Candida
sepsis (burn wounds)	Pseudomonas aeruginosa
diarrhea - children **- adults (US)** **- travelers**	**- Rotavirus** **- Campylobacter** **- E. coli, shigella, salmonella**
genital ulcer	herpes > syphilis
urethritis	chlamydia > gonococcus
cystitis	E. coli

Part B : Bacteria

2.7.) STAPHYLOCOCCI
(catalase +)

	coagulase	novobiocin	diseases
S. aureus	+		skin infections osteomyelitis endocarditis toxic shock syndrome food poisoning
S. epidermidis	-	sensitive	infections following: instrumentation implants etc.
S. saprophyticus	-	insensitive	urinary tract infections

Famous exotoxins:
- Enterotoxin A-F -> diarrhea
- Toxic shock syndrome toxin -> anaphylaxis
- Exfoliatin -> scalded skin (hands and feet)
- Alpha toxin ->tissue necrosis

Staph. aureus:
- *colonizes anterior nares of most people.*
- *community cases usually due to poor hygiene.*
- *hospital cases usually involve patients who underwent invasive procedures.*
- *survives drying! Often spread by hands of medical personnel.*

2.8.) STREPTOCOCCI
(catalase -)

Compared to staphylococci : - grow better on enriched medium
- narrower temperature range
- in culture: small colonies, no pigment

	key features
ß-hemolytic streptococci complete hemolysis (clear halo)	**Strept. pyogenes (Group A)**[1] - pharyngitis - acute rheumatic fever - bacitracin sensitive **other Strept. (Groups B-T)**[1] - neonatal sepsis - meningitis - bacitracin insensitive

[1] C-antigen, cell-wall, determines group (=Lancefield antigen)

"Strep throat":
- *acute sore throat*
- *malaise, fever (39⁰ - 40⁰)*
- *yellow exudates on tonsils*
- *may need bacterial culture to distinguish from viral pharyngitis*

	key features
α-hemolytic streptococci incomplete hemolysis (green halo)	**Pneumococci** - lobar pneumonia - capsule determines virulence (over 80 distinct serotypes) - bile soluble (lysis) - Optochin sensitive **Strept. viridans** - endocarditis - bile insoluble - Optochin insensitive
γ-hemolytic streptococci no hemolysis	**Enterococci (Group D)**[1] - urinary tract infections

 Enterococci are more resistant to antibiotics than other streptococci.

Famous exotoxins:
- Streptokinase
- Streptodornase (DNAse)
- Hyaluronidase
- Erythrogenic toxin
- Streptolysin O
- Streptolysin S

2.9.)   NEISSERIA
(gram-negative diplococci)

	key features
Meningococcus	- has capsule - ferments maltose - meningitis (infants 6-24 months) [1] - Waterhouse-Friderichsen syndrome - Gram stain of CSF is diagnostic - *TX: penicillin G*

Gonococcus	- has pilus
	- does not ferment maltose
	
	- **male** : dysuria, purulent discharge
	- **female**: endocervical infections
	                 salpingitis
	                 infertility
	
	- *TX: ceftriaxone is drug of choice*
	          (plus tetracycline for coexisting
	             C. trachomatis infection)

[1] "natural immunity" in first 6 months of life due to maternal IgG (transplacental)

Always suspect gonorrhea in adolescents and young adults with purulent arthritis (common !)

2.10.) <u>BACILLI</u>

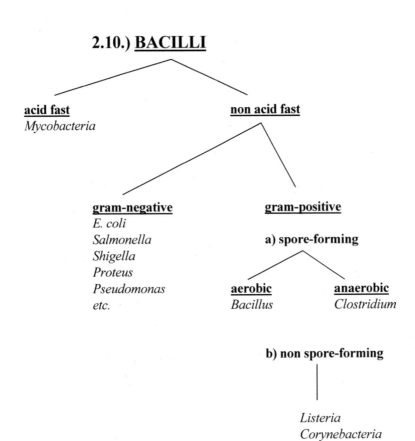

<u>acid fast</u>
Mycobacteria

<u>non acid fast</u>

<u>gram-negative</u>
E. coli
Salmonella
Shigella
Proteus
Pseudomonas
etc.

<u>gram-positive</u>

a) spore-forming

<u>aerobic</u>
Bacillus

<u>anaerobic</u>
Clostridium

b) non spore-forming

Listeria
Corynebacteria

94

2.11.) <u>GRAM-POSITIVE BACILLI</u>

	aerobe	toxins	spores	
Bacillus anthracis	+	+	+	- anthrax - woolsorter's disease - "fried rice" poisoning

Coryne-bacterium	+	+	-	- diphtheria
				  pseudomembranes
				  Loeffler's telluride
				  "Chinese characters"

Listeria	+	-	-	- sepsis, meningitis - neonates or immunosuppressed - "Chinese characters" + motile!
Clostridium	-	+	+	- tetanus - botulism - gas gangrene (α-toxin) - food poisoning (reheated meat) - pseudomembranous colitis
Lactobacillus	-	-	-	- protects GI and vagina - prefers acidic pH < 4.5

<u>**Pseudomembranous colitis:**</u>
(most common offending antibiotics)
- clindamycin
- ampicillin
- cephalosporins

2.12.) CLOSTRIDIA

	key features
Cl. botulinum	- non-capsulate, sporing, motile - types A-G (antigenically different exotoxins)
Cl. tetani	- non-capsulate, sporing, motile - 10 types (flagellar antigen) - but all have the same exotoxin
Cl. perfringens	- non-capsulate, sporing, non-motile - α-toxin = lecithinase causes gas gangrene (soldiers) - enterotoxin (heat labile) causes food poisoning (reheated meat stews)

BOTULISM:
- *Cl. Botulinum* spores are highly resistant to heat, but toxins are not.
- Proper canning and heating of food prevents botulism.
- Nausea, vomiting and abdominal cramps usually precede the neurological symptoms: Dry mouth, diplopia, loss of pupillary reflexes, followed by descending paralysis and respiratory failure.

TETANUS:
- Toxin enters the CNS along the peripheral nerves
- Incubation period 5 to 10 days
- Stiffness of the jaws, difficulty swallowing, fever, headache
- *Risus sardonicus*: fixed "smile" and elevated eyebrows
- Severe spasms of neck, back and abdominal muscles
- Intact sensorium and CSF

2.13.) <u>ENTEROBACTERIACEAE</u>
(facultative anaerobe, glucose + oxidase -)

Gram negative bacilli. 5 major genera. All look the same, some are motile, some are not. Differentiated by cultural appearance and biochemical activities. Subtyping is done by serology.

	lab features	clinical features
E. coli	motile lactose + indole -	- most common cause of UTI - neonatal meningitis [1]
Salmonella (1,500 species)	motile lactose - indole - only *S. typhi* produces gas	**food poisoning** - poultry products - incubation 1-2 days **enteric fever (typhoid, paratyphoid)** - incubation 10-14 days
Shigella	non-motile lactose - indole + no gas	**dysenteriae** (serious) **flexneri, boydii, sonnei** (mild) - watery diarrhea followed by fever, bloody stools and cramping

[1] maternal IgM does NOT cross placenta -> no protection

Shigella is 1,000x more infective than Salmonella.

<u>TREATMENT OF SALMONELLA INFECTIONS:</u>
gastroenteritis: fluid replacement, no antibiotics
typhoid: chloramphenicol, ampicillin

	lab features	clinical features
Proteus [1]	motile (swarms !) urease	**urinary tract infections** urease-production -> ammonium calculi proteus does NOT cause gastroenteritis
Klebsiella	non-motile lactose + produces slime (M antigen)	**lobar pneumonia** - "currant jelly" sputum - resistant to many antibiotics!

[1] has antigens that cross-react with anti-rickettsial antibodies
(Weil-Felix reaction)

> *K-antigen*: *capsule*
> *H-antigen*: *flagella*
> *O-antigen*: *surface*

2.14.) <u>MORE ENTEROBACTERIACEAE</u>

	key features
Bacteroides fragilis	- most common cause of gram-negative abdominal infections - anaerobic, likes bile - forms abscess - *TX: metronidazole*
Vibrio cholera	- rice-watery diarrhea (non bloody) - comma shaped - *TX: tetracycline*
Vibrio parahaemolyticus	- diarrhea from raw or uncooked seafood (sushi) - *self-limited*
Campylobacter jejuni	- watery, foul smelling stools later may become bloody - very common in US - grows best at 5% CO_2, 42°C - *TX: erythromycin, aminoglycoside*
Helicobacter pylori	- a/w gastritis and peptic ulcer - very similar to Campylobacter (but urease +) - *TX: metronidazole + tetracycline + bismuth*

2.15.) GRAM-NEGATIVE BACILLI (ZOONOTIC)

	key features
Yersinia pestis	- **bubonic plague** rodents -> fleas -> humans large, very tender lymph nodes - **pulmonary plague** humans -> humans - *TX: streptomycin, tetracycline*
Pasteurella	- bipolar staining - wound infections (dog and cat bites) - cellulitis, osteomyelitis - *TX: penicillin G*
Brucella	- undulating fever - Br. abortus (placentitis in cows) - Br. melitensis (goats and sheep) - Br. suis (pigs) - *TX: tetracycline, gentamycin*
Francisella	- tularemia - rabbits -> ticks -> humans - influenza like, adenopathy - *TX: streptomycin*

Plague ("Black Death") killed 25 million people in Europe in the 14th Century. Today, 30-40 cases/year are reported in the US. Bubonic plague has up to 75% mortality, pneumonic plague has 100% mortality if untreated. Avoid sick or dead wild rodents!

2.16.) OTHER GRAM-NEGATIVE BACILLI

	key features
Pseudomonas	- does not ferment glucose - oxidase + - musty odor, greenish bluish pus - common wound infection (especially burns) - pneumonia, UTI - *resists most antibiotics and disinfectants*
Hemophilus	- requires blood (chocolate agar) - requires coagulation factors V and X - grows around staphylococci (satellites) - **H. influenza** : bronchitis, meningitis - **H. ducreyi** : chancroid - H. hemolyticus : may be confused with S. pyogenes (but is gram - and resists bacitracin)
Bordetella	- pertussis toxin -> whooping cough - diagnosis: nasopharyngeal swab plated on charcoal blood agar - *TX: erythromycin (best during catarrhal stage!)*
Legionella	- gram-negative cell wall, but stains only faintly - atypical pneumonia - no cold agglutinins (unlike mycoplasma) - grows in water reservoirs - *TX: erythromycin*

***Whooping cough**: catarrhal stage (1-2 weeks): rhinorrhea, malaise, fever*
coughing stage (2-4 weeks): up to 50 episodes per day!

2.17.) MYCOBACTERIA

	key features
M. tuberculosis	- slow respiratory infection - primary lesion: **Ghon complex** - most morbidity is due to reactivation
M. bovis	- unpasteurized milk - GI tuberculosis

M. leprae	- prefers 32°C (rather than 37°C)
	- found in nasal secretions and skin lesions
	- **tuberculoid leprosy**: granulomas
	                 skin test positive
	- **lepromatous leprosy**: nodular skin lesions
	                 skin test negative

Atypical	
M. marinum	- swimming pool granuloma
M. avium-intracellulare	- clinically indistinguishable from tuberculosis - highly resistant to therapy - immunosuppressed patients (AIDS!)
M. fortuitum	- saprophyte - rapidly growing - highly resistant to therapy

	TUBERCULOSIS:
Ghon complex:	primary lesion in lung plus calcified hilar lymph node
reactivation:	favors upper lobes of lung liquefying necrosis -> cavity formation
miliary TBC:	due to hematogenous spread of tubercle bacilli (lesions resemble millet seeds)

2.18.) HIGHER BACTERIA

- gram-positive rods
- filamentous, branching growth, were confused with fungi in the past
- cause indolent, slowly progressive diseases

	key features
Actinomyces	- anaerobe - growths in normal mouth flora **Lump jaw** - following tooth extraction - inflammatory sinuses -> discharge to surface - sulfur granules *TX: penicillin* * surgical drainage*
Nocardia	- aerobe - growths in soil **Subcutaneous tissue infections** - following minor trauma (outdoors) **Pulmonary infections** - inhalation of dust or soil *TX: sulfonamides* * surgical drainage*

2.19.) <u>SPIROCHETES</u>

	key features
T. pallidum	- syphilis - related diseases: Yaws, Bejel, Pinta - *TX: penicillin G*
B. burgdorferi	- Lyme disease - tick bite (mainly east coast) - *TX: acute: tetracycline* *chronic: penicillin G*
B. recurrentis	- relapsing fever - antigens undergo variations -> relapses - human -> louse -> human - *TX: tetracycline*
L. interrogans	- leptospirosis - sewers, water contaminated with rat urine - fever, jaundice, hemorrhage, uremia - *TX: penicillin G*

<u>LYME DISEASE</u>:

1.) primary lesion (3-30 days): - at site of tick bite
- expanding macule or papule with
central clearing *(erythema migrans)*
2.) second stage (weeks - months): - cardiac AV block
- fluctuating meningitis
- facial palsy
- peripheral neuropathy
3.) third stage (weeks - years): - arthritis of large joints (knee)

2.20.) CHLAMYDIA

	key features
C. pneumoniae	- "walking pneumonia" in young adults - *TX: tetracycline*

C. trachomatis	**different strains cause different diseases :**
	
	- **urethritis**
	  most common non-gonorrheal urethritis
	
	- **lymphogranuloma venereum**
	  purulent, but often asymptomatic in male
	
	- **trachoma**
	  chronic conjunctivitis that leads to blindness
	
	- *TX: tetracycline*

C. psittaci	- **pneumonia**, sometimes with hepatitis - from bird feces - *TX: tetracycline*

 Giemsa stain shows typical cytoplasmic inclusions in epithelial cells.

Life cycle of chlamydiae:
- elementary body infects cell (attaches to cell membrane)
- enters cells by endocytosis
- elementary body transforms to large reticulate body
  (visible cytoplasmic inclusions)
- reticulate body condenses and forms many new elementary bodies
- new elementary bodies are released when cell ruptures

2.21.) <u>RICKETTSIA</u>

		vector	reservoir
Typhus: epidemic [1] **endemic** [2] **scrub** [3]	*R. prowazekii* *R. typhi* *R. tsutsugamushi*	lice fleas mite	humans rodents rodents
Rocky Mountain spotted fever	*R. rickettsiae*	ticks	dogs, rodents
Q fever	*C. burnetii*	transmitted by inhalation (slaughterhouses)	cattle, sheep
Trench fever	*R. quintana*	lice	humans

 Treatment of rickettsial infections: tetracycline

[1] war, famine, crowding, infrequent bathing (no cases in US since WW II)
[2] murine typhus, 30-60 cases/year in US (mainly Texas)
[3] Southeast Asia, Japan

Part C : Viruses

2.22.) DNA VIRUSES

- all have double stranded genome except parvovirus
- all are icosahedral except poxvirus

family	virus	diseases
Parvo	B19	- erythema infectiosum, (5th disease) "slapped cheek"
Papova	Papilloma	- genital warts -> cervix carcinoma - multiply in squamous cells
	JC	- leukoencephalopathy (immunocompromised patients)
Adeno	~100 serotypes	- respiratory infections - atypical pneumonia - conjunctivitis - gastroenteritis - hemorrhagic cystitis
Pox	Variola	- smallpox
	Vaccinia	- cowpox
	Molluscum contagiosum	- small pink warts, benign
Hepadna	HBV	- serum hepatitis B - liver cell carcinoma

Vaccinia is serologically related to Variola, but the origin of this virus (recombinant of smallpox and cowpox?) is unknown.

2.23.) <u>HERPES VIRUSES</u>
(double stranded DNA)

virus	diseases	during latency the virus rests in:
HSV1 **HSV2**	- mainly oral herpes - mainly genital herpes - both multiply in fibroblasts	trigeminal ganglion sacral DRG
VZV	- chickenpox, shingles	thoracolumbar DRG [1]
EBV	- infectious mononucleosis - Burkitt's lymphoma (Africa) - nasopharyngeal carcinoma (China)	B lymphocytes
CMV	- cytomegalic inclusion disease - heterophil negative mononucleosis (no pharyngitis !)	leukocytes
HHV-6	- roseola (6th disease)	T lymphocytes
HHV-7	- unknown	unknown

[1] *DRG = dorsal root ganglion: eruptions follow sensory nerve distribution!*

Chickenpox: lesions appear in <u>different</u> stages of evolution
(vesicular -> pustular -> crusts)
Smallpox: lesions appear in <u>same</u> stage of evolution

2.24.) RNA VIRUSES

family	virus	diseases
Picorna	Hepatitis A Polio	- infectious hepatitis A - paralysis (α-motoneuron)
	Coxsackie A Coxsackie B	- herpangina - hand/foot/mouth disease - myocarditis - Bornholm disease
	Echo Rhino	- meningitis, URI, diarrhea - common cold
Reo	Rota	- gastroenteritis (children)
Orthomyxo	Influenza A, B, C	- influenza
Paramyxo	**Rubeola**	- measles - encephalitis - SSPE
	Mumps RSV Parainfluenza	- parotitis, orchitis - bronchiolitis, pneumonia - croup (subglottitis)
Toga	**Rubella** Arbo	- German measles - encephalitis (arthropod vectors)

Antigenic shift:	- subtle changes of H or N antigen - due to single mutation of viral RNA - occurs every few years
Antigenic drift:	- major, sudden change of H and/or N antigens - due to recombination of genes - occurs every 8-10 years -> severe epidemics

2.25.) <u>ARBO VIRUSES</u>
(arthropod borne)

family	virus	diseases	vector
Toga	**Alphavirus**	- EEE - WEE	mosquito
Flavi	**Flavivirus**	- St. Louis encephalitis - yellow fever - Dengue fever	mosquito
Bunya	**Bunyavirus**	- California encephalitis	mosquito
	Hantavirus	- fulminant respiratory infection	deer mice
Reo	**Orbivirus**	- Colorado tick fever	tick

 Hantavirus is an exception among Arboviruses: no arthropod vector!

2.26.) <u>SLOW VIRAL DISEASES OF CNS</u>

Progressive neurologic diseases due to viral persistence.

- personality changes
- intellectual deterioration
- autonomic or motor dysfunctions

AIDS dementia complex	HIV
subacute sclerosing panencephalitis	measles virus
progressive multifocal leukoencephalopathy	JC virus

2.27.) <u>PRIONS</u>

<u>Prions are infectious proteins</u> :
- can be transmitted to other species (chimpanzees, mice etc.) by inoculation of infected brain tissue
- are NOT transmitted by body secretions (-> no risk for medical personnel and care givers)
- are NOT inactivated by formalin!

kuru ("trembling disease")	prions
Creutzfeldt-Jakob	prions
scrapie	prions
bovine spongiform encephalopathy	prions

2.28.) <u>RETROVIRUSES</u>

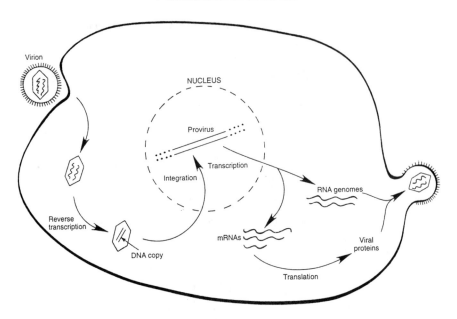

From *Sherris Medical Microbiology*, 3rd edition, p. 544, edited by Kenneth J. Ryan.
Copyright 1994 by Appleton&Lange, Norwalk, Connecticut. Used with permission.

oncoviruses	HTLV-1	adult T-cell leukemia
lentiviruses	HIV-1 HIV-2	AIDS

HTLV-1 simply activates existing cellular genes (c-onc = protooncogenes) resulting in malignant transformation.

Other retroviruses cause tumors (in animals) by expressing viral oncogenes (v-onc) or inserting promoters or enhancers in the vicinity of proto-oncogenes (c-onc).

2.29.) <u>HIV</u>

genome	- two identical single strands of RNA (positive polarity)
gag	- internal core protein: p24 (serologic marker)
pol	- reverse transcriptase - integrase - protease
env	- gp: glycoproteins in lipid envelope **- gp41 : mediates cell fusion** **- gp120 : binds to CD4 receptor** (mutates rapidly !)
tat	- regulatory gene - increases rate of transcription - also suppresses synthesis of class I MHC proteins

> ***ELISA (screening):*** *very sensitive*
>   *fairly specific*
>
> ***Western blot:***   *very specific*
>   *done to confirm a positive ELISA*

 Antibodies are not detectable for 2-4 weeks after infection.

Part D : Fungi & Parasites

2.30.) FUNGI

WHAT THEY LOOK LIKE:

*Fungi come it two forms : **Yeasts** (single cells) and **Molds** (forming hyphae) Most fungi can be both (i.e. are dimorphic). Typically they form yeasts at 37°C and molds if they grow outside the human body.*

EXAMPLES:

MOLDS	DIMORPHIC FUNGI	YEASTS
- **aspergillus** farmer's lung	- **histoplasma** pulmonary infection	- **candida** thrush, vaginitis
	- **blastomyces** respiratory tract infection	- **cryptococcus** pneumonia, meningitis
	- **coccidioides** desert rheumatism	

MOLDS:

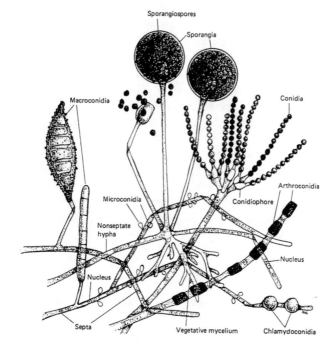

Sporangiospores
Sporangia
Macroconidia
Conidia
Microconidia
Arthroconidia
Conidiophore
Nonseptate hypha
Nucleus
Nucleus
Septa
Vegetative mycelium
Chlamydoconidia

YEASTS:

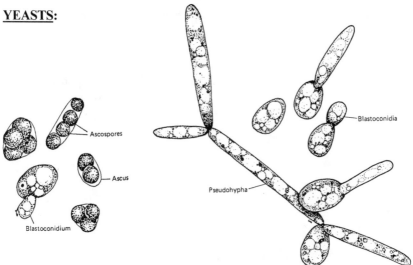

Ascospores
Ascus
Blastoconidium
Blastoconidia
Pseudohypha

From *Sherris Medical Microbiology*, 3rd edition, p. 574, edited by Kenneth J. Ryan.
Copyright 1994 by Appleton&Lange, Norwalk, Connecticut. Used with permission.

HOW THEY REPRODUCE:

Fungi reproduce in two manners : Sexual and asexual.
Most fungi can do both (i.e. fungi perfecti).
Fungi that do not reproduce sexually are called fungi imperfecti.
(or maybe they "couple" so rarely, that their spores went undetected so far)

- **Sexual reproduction:** 2 cells fuse, diploid cell divides by meiosis
- **Asexual reproduction:** haploid cell divides by mitosis (like bacteria)

---

spores (sexual): Ascospores, Basidiospores, Zygospores etc.
conidia (asexual): Arthroconidia, Chlamydioconidia etc.

Note how both yeasts and molds can produce spores and conidia:

	yeasts	molds
asexual	Blastoconidia (="buds") Pseudohyphae	Arthroconidia Chlamydioconidia
sexual	Ascospores	Basidiospores Zygospores

2.31.) FUNGAL DISEASES

		microscopic features
cutaneous	- **dermatophytosis** [1] (ringworm) - **tinea versicolor**	- hyphae - hyphae
subcutaneous	- **mycetoma** - **sporotrichosis**	- "tree" shaped (sporangia) - cigar shaped budding yeast
systemic	- **coccidioidomycosis** - **histoplasmosis** - **blastomycosis**	- soil: arthrospores tissue: endospores - yeasts in macrophages - broad based bud with double refractory walls
opportunistic	- **cryptococcosis** - **candidiasis** - **aspergillosis**	- capsule on India ink prep. - pseudohyphae germ tubes - V shaped

> ***Diagnosis** by light microscopy : 10% KOH prep (dissolves tissue but not fungal wall)*

Histoplasmosis:- humid soil (Mississippi river)
- most infections are asymptomatic
- progressive pulmonary disease resembles tuberculosis

Coccidioidomycosis: - "valley fever": fever, cough, arthralgia
- endemic to Arizona, Nevada, New Mexico.

Aspergillosis: - allergy, exacerbates asthma
- pulmonary disease (immunocompromised patients)
- radiologically visible fungus ball within cavity

117

2.32.) MALARIA

Mosquito :	**sexual cycle ->**	forms sporozoites
Human :	**asexual cycle ->**	forms schizonts

1.) **Sporozoites** are introduced into blood
2.) Exo-erythrocytic phase: sporozoites differentiate into merozoites
3.) **Merozoites** settle in liver (latent forms called hypnozoites)
4.) Liver releases merozoites
5.) Merozoites infect red blood cells
6.) Ring-shaped **trophozoite** matures, forms multinucleated schizonts
7.) RBC releases either 10-20 new merozoites **or gametocytes**

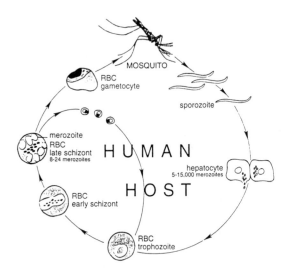

From *Sherris Medical Microbiology*, 3rd edition, p. 644, edited by Kenneth J. Ryan.
Copyright 1994 by Appleton&Lange, Norwalk, Connecticut. Used with permission.

	key features
Vivax	- fever peak every 48 h - latent liver forms
Ovale	- fever peak every 48 h - latent liver forms
Falciparum	- fever peak every 48 h - most severe, life threatening - no trophozoites/schizonts found in blood - banana shaped gametocytes
Malariae	- fever peak every 72 h

Prevention:
- mosquito screens, repellents
- mefloquine or doxycycline when traveling to areas where chloroquine-resistance is common

2.33.) <u>TISSUE PROTOZOA</u>

Pneumocystis carinii	- probably a fungus, (but antifungal drugs are ineffective!) - common in **AIDS** patients - sudden onset fever, dyspnea, tachypnea - *TX: trimethoprim-sulfamethoxazole* *pentamidine*
Toxoplasma gondii	- cat feces, undercooked meat (pork) - ingestion: cysts -> invade gut wall - differentiate into trophozoites (tachyzoites) - tachyzoites may **invade brain**, muscle and form slowly growing cysts (bradyzoites) - *TX: sulfonamide (first trimester)* *sulfonamide-pyrimethamine (all others)*
Leishmania a) L. donovani b) L. brasiliensis c) L. mexicana, L. tropica	 a) Kala-Azar (**visceral**) "black sickness" (GI bleeding) b) Espundia (**mucocutaneous ulcers**) c) **cutaneous** leishmaniosis (red papule, satellites, ulcerating) - *TX: sodium stibogluconate*
Trypanosoma a) T. cruzi b) T. gambiense c) T. rhodesiense	 a) American trypanosomiasis (Chagas disease) - kissing bug - *TX: nifurtimox* b) Tsetse fly : African sleeping sickness c) more severe than T. gambiense - *TX: suramin, melarsoprol*

2.34.) <u>INTESTINAL PROTOZOA</u>

Entamoeba histolytica	- cysts have 4 nuclei - bloody, mucus, diarrhea - liver abscess - can be sexually transmitted - *TX: metronidazole*
Giardia lamblia	- cyst: 4 nuclei - trophozoite: 2 nuclei, 4 pairs of flagella (looks like a clown....) - excystation in duodenum - non-bloody, foul smelling diarrhea - *TX: metronidazole*
Cryptosporidium	- excystation in small intestine - trophozoites do not invade gut wall - severe diarrhea in immunocompromised (AIDS!) - *no effective therapy*

<u>ANOTHER PROTOZOON JUST FOR COMPARISON:</u>

Trichomonas	- 1 nucleus, 4 flagella, undulating membrane - **most common VD in the US !** - male : non-purulent urethritis (often asymptomatic) - female: foul-smelling, watery, green discharge - *TX: metronidazole*

2.35.) <u>TREMATODES (FLUKES)</u>

	route of infection:	eventually settles in:
Sch. mansoni	penetrates skin	veins of colon
Sch. japonicum	penetrates skin	veins of small intestine
Sch. hematobium	penetrates skin	veins of urinary bladder
Clonorchis sinensis	raw fish	liver
Paragonimus	raw crab meat	lung

TX: Praziquantel works for all flukes.

2.36.) <u>CESTODES (TAPEWORMS)</u>

	source	ingested form	eventually settles in:
T. solium	pork	larvae	intestine
T. solium	human feces	eggs	cysticerci (in brain, eyes)
T. saginata	beef	larvae	intestine
D. latum	raw fish	larvae	intestine
Echinococcus	dog feces	eggs	cysts (in liver, lung, brain)

TX: Niclosamide works for all tapeworms.

2.37.) <u>NEMATODES (ROUNDWORMS)</u>

<u>INGESTED FORM: EGGS</u>

Enterobius	perianal pruritus (at night)
Ascaris	worm lives in colon, larvas migrate to lung

<u>INGESTED FORM: LARVAE</u>

Necator	intestinal blood loss
Strongyloides	larvas penetrate skin, then migrate to lung
Trichinella	pork meat, larvae form cysts in striated muscle

<u>TRANSMITTED BY INSECT BITE</u>:

Wuchereria	microfilariae found in blood adult worm lives in lymph nodes -> lymph obstruction
Onchocerca	"river blindness" microfilariae in subcutaneous tissue and eye

PHARMACOLOGY

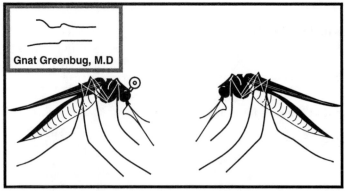

"Chemotherapy will increase your lifespan about 10 minutes, Mr. Mosley, which is not bad, given your normal life cycle of 2 days."

3.1.) <u>DRUG INTERACTIONS</u>

drugs that are easily displaced from albumins	sulfonamides phenylbutazone tolbutamide coumarin
drugs that induce P450	alcohol barbiturates phenytoin rifampicin
drugs that inhibit P450	chloramphenicol sulfonamides phenylbutazone
drugs that compete for renal transporters	(uric acid) probenecid penicillins sulfonamides salicylates thiazides

EXAMPLES:

(1) Risk of severe hemorrhage if coumarins are combined with any other drug that competes for albumin.

(2) Sulfonamides displace sulfonylureas from albumin → hypoglycemia

(3) Barbiturate induces P450 enzyme → enhanced metabolism of MAO inhibitors → ineffective treatment of depression.

(4) P450 induction → Enhanced estrogen metabolism → reduced oral contraceptive efficacy → unplanned pregnancy

(5) Steroids compete with MAO inhibitor for P450 enzyme → reduced metabolism of MAO inhibitor → risk of over dose

(6) Aspirin reduces renal secretion of uric acid and is contraindicated in gout.

3.2.) **BAD COMBINATIONS**

never ever combine:	with these drugs:
aminoglycosides	neuromuscular blockers (enhanced block) loop diuretics (compounds ototoxicity)
MAO inhibitors	levodopa (hypertensive crisis) amphetamine (hypertensive crisis) tricyclic antidepressants [1]
tricyclic antidepressants	MAO inhibitors [1]

[1] antidepressants should never be combined!

3.3.) <u>FAMOUS SIDE EFFECTS</u>

famous side effect:	caused by:
anaphylactic shock	- penicillin - foreign proteins
hepatotoxicity	- isoniazid - halothane
renal toxicity	- phenacetin - other NSAIDs - cyclosporin
ototoxicity	- aminoglycosides
drug-induced lupus	- procainamide - hydralazine
photosensitivity (skin)	- tetracyclines - sulfonamides - sulfonylureas
cutaneous flushing	- niacin
hemolysis in patients with G6PD-deficiency	- sulfonamides - primaquine
bone marrow suppression	- chloramphenicol - ganciclovir - zidovudine (AZT)

3.4.) ANTIDOTES

intoxication	antidote
acetaminophen	N-acetylcysteine
opiates	naloxone
benzodiazepines	flumazenil
methanol, ethylene glycol	ethanol
CO	100% O_2
cyanide	amyl nitrate
organophosphates	atropine, pralidoxime
iron	deferoxamine
lead	EDTA
coumarins	Vit. K
heparin	protamine

Intoxication with acidic drugs (e.g. barbiturate, salicylate):
Alkalinize urine (IV sodium-bicarbonate) to enhance renal excretion.

3.5.) ANTIBIOTICS

- **Bactericidal** drugs "kill" bacteria.
- **Bacteriostatic** drugs inhibit bacterial growth and require the host's immune system to "finish the job".

bactericidal	bacteriostatic
penicillins	chloramphenicol
cephalosporins	erythromycin
aminoglycosides	tetracyclines
vancomycin	sulfonamides
	trimethoprim

 Misuse of antibiotics results in emergence of antibiotic-resistant strains. This creates an ever-increasing need for new drugs.

gram-positive	gram-negative	broad-spectrum
penicillin G	aminoglycosides	ampicillin
vancomycin	polymyxins	cephalosporins
bacitracin		tetracyclines
		chloramphenicol
		sulfonamides

MECHANISMS OF RESISTANCE:

transduction	bacteriophages that carry plasmids (extrachromosomal DNA)
transformation	uptake and incorporation of DNA from environment
conjugation	direct transmission of DNA from cell to cell via sex pilus

3.6.) <u>DRUGS OF CHOICE</u>

Actinomyces	actinomycosis	penicillin G
Bacillus anthracis	anthrax	penicillin G
Bordetella pertussis	whooping cough	erythromycin
Borrelia Burgdorferi	Lyme disease	tetracycline
Campylobacter	acute inflammatory diarrhea	ciprofloxacin
Candida	vaginal candidiasis	miconazole
	systemic candidiasis	fluconazole
Chlamydia trachomatis	pelvic inflammatory disease	doxycycline
Chlamydia pneumoniae	pneumonia	tetracycline
H. influenza	pneumonia, meningitis	3rd gen. cephalosporin
Helicobacter pylori	gastric ulcer	metronidazole + tetracycline
Klebsiella	pneumonia	3rd gen. cephalosporin
	UTI	quinolones
Legionella	Legionnaire's disease	erythromycin
M. tuberculosis	tuberculosis	isoniazid + rifampin
		+ pyrazinamide + ethambutol
M. leprae	leprosy	dapsone + rifampin
M. pneumoniae	atypical pneumonia	erythromycin
N. gonorrhea	gonorrhea	ceftriaxone
N. meningitis	meningitis	penicillin G
Nocardia	pneumonia	trimethoprim/sulfamethoxazole
Proteus	UTI	quinolones
Rickettsia	spotted fever, end. typhus	tetracycline
Salmonella typhi	typhoid fever	trimethoprim/sulfamethoxazole
Shigella	dysentery	trimethoprim/sulfamethoxazole
Staph. aureus	skin infection	dicloxacillin
	sepsis, osteomyelitis	nafcillin or oxacillin
Strept. pyogenes	pharyngitis, erysipelas	penicillin G or V
Strept. viridans	endocarditis	penicillin + aminoglycoside
Treponema pallidum	syphilis	penicillin G
Trichomonas	trichomoniasis	metronidazole
Tropheryma whippelii	Whipple's disease	trimethoprim/sulfamethoxazole
Vibrio cholerae	cholera	tetracycline (+ fluids!)
Yersinia pestis	plague ("black death")	streptomycin

3.7.) PENICILLINS

narrow spectrum β-lactamase sensitive	penicillin G penicillin V	gram positive *Strept.*
β-lactamase resistant	methicillin oxacillin nafcillin cloxacillin	gram positive *Strept.*
broad spectrum	ampicillin amoxicillin	*Hemophilus* *Neisseria* *E. coli* *Proteus*
extended spectrum	carbenicillin	*Pseudomonas*

SIDE-EFFECTS:
- Allergic reactions (maculopapular rash)
  Cross-reactivity with cephalosporins!
- Diarrhea (disruption of normal flora)

β-LACTAMASE (arrow indicates site of action):

penicillin   cephalosporin

3.8.) CEPHALOSPORINS

1st Generation (against gram-positive plus E. coli, Klebsiella)

cefazolin	longest half life
cephalexin	acid stable (oral administration)

2nd Generation (broader spectrum against gram-negative bacilli)

cefamandole	☹ disulfiram like reaction with ethanol bleeding (anti vitamin K action)
cefoxitin	potent against anaerobes (bowel perforation -> E. coli, Bacteroides fragilis)

3rd Generation (superior activity against enterobacteriaceae)

cefotaxime	CNS permeable (Hemophilus meningitis!)
ceftriaxone	drug of choice for penicillin resistant gonorrhea

☹

SIDE-EFFECTS:
- Avoid in patients with known penicillin allergy. (significant cross reactivity)

3.9.) ANTIVIRAL DRUGS

	mechanism of action	used to treat
amantadine	impairs uncoating	influenza A
ribavirin	guanosine analog	RSV infections in children
acyclovir	guanine analog, depends on viral thymidine kinase	HSV-1, HSV-2, VZV
vidarabine	adenosine analog	all Herpes group viruses
idoxuridine	thymidine analog	Herpes simplex keratitis
ganciclovir	like acyclovir	CMV
AZT	thymidine analog	HIV
interferon	inhibits viral multiplication	leukemia Kaposi sarcoma genital warts hepatitis B and C

AZT: 3'-azido-3'-deoxythymidine

3.10.) <u>ANTIFUNGAL DRUGS</u>

systemic fungal infections	amphotericin B, ketoconazole
candida and skin infections	nystatin
broad spectrum anti-fungals	imidazoles
dermatophytic Infections	griseofulvin (accumulates in keratin)

> **<u>SIDE-EFFECTS</u>:**
> - **Griseofulvin:** hepatotoxic, teratogenic
> - **Amphotericin:** nephrotoxic, anemia
> - **Nystatin, miconazole:** systemic toxicity
> used only topically

3.11.) ANTI-PROTOZOAL DRUGS

MALARIA:

prophylaxis	mefloquine
therapy	chloroquine
therapy (P. falciparum)	quinine + pyrimethamine/sulfadoxine
prevention of relapse	primaquine [1]

[1] eradicates persistent liver stages (*P. vivax* and *P. ovale*)

OTHER PROTOZOA:

amebiasis (*Trichomonas, Chlamydia*)	metronidazole
leishmaniasis	stibogluconate
African sleeping sickness *(Trypanosoma gambiense)* *(Trypanosoma rhodesiense)*	melarsoprol / suramin
Chagas disease *(Trypanosoma cruzi)*	nifurtimox

3.12.) <u>AIDS</u>

<u>HIV:</u>

1st line of drugs	nucleoside analogs: zidovudine (AZT) ± didanosine [1]
add next	protease inhibitors
experimental	non-nucleotide reverse transcriptase inhibitors

[1] several other combinations are also possible

<u>OPPORTUNISTIC INFECTIONS:</u>

Herpes simplex or zoster	acyclovir
CMV	ganciclovir
M. avium complex	clarithromycin + ethambutol
Candida (esophageal)	fluconazole, ketoconazole
Cryptococcus neoformans	fluconazole
Pneumocystis carinii [1]	trimethoprim-sulfamethoxazole (pentamidine if allergic)
Toxoplasma gondii	pyrimethamine-sulfadiazine

[1] prophylaxis necessary if CD4 < 200/µL

3.13.) INHIBITORS OF TRANSLATION
RNA → Protein

PROKARYOTES:

	acts on:	mechanism of action
aminoglycosides	30 S	inhibits initiation (binding of tRNA$_{fm}$)
tetracyclines	30 S	inhibits binding of all other tRNAs
chloramphenicol	50 S	inhibits peptidyl transferase
erythromycin	50 S	inhibits translocation

EUKARYOTES:

	acts on:	mechanism of action:
lectins	40/60 S	inhibits initiation
cycloheximide	60 S	inhibits peptidyl transferase
diphtheria toxin	60 S	inhibits elongation factor

Puromycin: - incorporated into peptide chain -> premature chain termination
- acts in both eukaryotes and prokaryotes
(not useful as antibiotic)

138

3.14.) <u>INHIBITORS OF REPLICATION</u>
DNA → DNA
<u>ANTI-FOLATES:</u>

	mechanism of action	clinical use
methotrexate	mammalian folate synthesis	anticancer drug
trimethoprim	bacterial folate synthesis	antibiotic
pyrimethamine	protozoal folate synthesis	antimalarial

<u>PURINE ANALOGS:</u>

mercaptopurine	inhibits de novo synthesis	-
azathioprine	derivative of mercaptopurine	immunosuppressant

<u>PYRIMIDINE ANALOGS:</u>

cytarabine (ara-CTP)	incorporated into DNA	anticancer drug
fluorouracil	inhibits thymidylate synthesis	anticancer drug

<u>ANTIBIOTICS:</u>

actinomycin D	binds to DNA	anticancer drug
doxorubicin	intercalates between base pairs	anticancer drug
bleomycin	causes strand breaks in DNA	anticancer drug

3.15.) <u>INHIBITORS OF TRANSCRIPTION</u>

rifampicin	- binds to bacterial DNA-dependent RNA polymerase inhibits initiation of RNA synthesis anti-tuberculosis
α-amanitin	- blocks eukaryotic polymerase II mushroom poison

actinomycin D	- binds to DNA
	  inhibits transcription (low concentration)
	  inhibits replication (high concentration)
	
	anticancer drug

doxorubicin	- intercalates between base pairs inhibits translation and replication anticancer drug
streptodigin	- inhibits elongation of prokaryotic RNA synthesis

3.16.) <u>COMBINATION CHEMOTHERAPY</u>

"Famous combinations":

ALL	prednisone
	vincristine
Wilms' tumor	dactinomycin
	vincristine
Hodgkin's disease	M mechlorethamine
	O vincristine
	P prednisone
	P procarbazine

😞 <u>SPECIFIC SIDE EFFECTS</u>:

doxorubicin	cardiotoxic
cyclophosphamide	hemorrhagic cystitis
bleomycin	pulmonary fibrosis
vincristine	peripheral neuropathy
cisplatin	renal toxicity
L-asparaginase	allergic reactions

> <u>*Cycle-specific drugs*</u> *:*
> *antimetabolites, bleomycin, vinca alkaloids*

3.17.) <u>NSAIDs</u>

<u>GENERAL USE NSAIDs:</u>

	mechanism of action	key features
aspirin	- acetylates cyclooxygenase	- analgesic: 600 mg/d - anti-inflammatory: 4g/d - may cause Reye's syndrome - contraindicated in gout !
acetaminophen	- no anti-inflammatory action - prefers CNS cyclooxygenase	- drug of choice for children with viral infections
ibuprofen	- similar spectrum as aspirin	- fewer GI side-effects
phenylbutazone	- anti-inflammatory - weak analgesic/antipyretic	- used when others have failed - may cause skin rash, GI upset
indomethacin	- more potent anti-inflammatory than aspirin	- for acute gout - for ankylosing spondylitis - may cause GI upset, pancreatitis

Aspirin: Acetylation of platelet cyclooxygenase is irreversible!
-> don't give within 1 week prior to surgery!
-> be careful with heparin!

> ### <u>SALICYLATE INTOXICATION:</u>
> - **mild**: tinnitus, central hyperventilation
> - **severe**: respiratory plus metabolic acidosis

NSAIDs FOR RHEUMATOID ARTHRITIS:

	mechanism of action	key features
gold	- suppresses macrophages	- for rheumatoid arthritis - not for acute attack
D-penicillamine	- reduces rheumatoid factor	- when gold has failed - also chelates heavy metals
methotrexate	- folic acid antagonist	- for severe rheumatoid arthritis [1] - when all else has failed ☹ may cause cytopenia

[1] much lower dose than when used for cancer therapy.

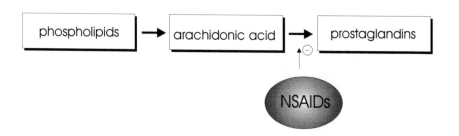

143

3.18.) <u>GOUT</u>

		mechanism of action
acute attack	**colchicine**	- inhibits migration of macrophages (depolymerizes microtubules) ☹ vomiting, abdominal pain
chronic gout	**allopurinol**	- purine analog - inhibits xanthine oxidase ☹ hypersensitivity reaction
chronic gout	**probenecid**	- blocks tubular secretion of penicillin [1] - blocks tubular reabsorption of uric acid

[1] occasionally used to increase serum levels of antibiotics.

Chronic gout: - elevated uric acid
- Lesch-Nyhan syndrome
- treatment of malignancies

3.19.) <u>ANTIHYPERTENSIVE DRUGS</u>

Choice of drug depends on clinical setting and contraindications:

	clinical setting	contraindications
β-blockers	- angina pectoris - post MI	- diabetes - asthma - peripheral vascular disease
thiazides	- congestive heart failure - chronic renal failure	- diabetes - hyperlipidemia
Ca^{2+} channel blockers	- for all patients	- congestive heart failure
ACE inhibitors	- for all patients	- pregnancy

 Hypertensive crisis: *Sodium nitroprusside acts rapidly!*

☹
> **SIDE-EFFECTS:**
> - **β-blockers**: - depression, fatigue, lethargy
>   - increases plasma triglycerides
> - **thiazides**: - hypokalemia
>   - hypercalcemia

3.20.) ANTI-ANGIOTENSINS

	key features
captopril	- ACE inhibitor - decreases angiotensin II - increases bradykinin
enalapril	- ACE inhibitor - more potent - longer half time
saralasin	- blocks angiotensin receptors (weak agonist)

ACE inhibitors work particularly well in young, white patients.

3.21.) ERGOT ALKALOIDS

	mechanism of action	indications
ergotamine, methysergide	vasoconstriction	- migraine - post partum hemorrhage
bromocriptine	inhibits prolactin release	- hyperprolactinemia (pituitary adenomas) - infertility

☹ diarrhea, nausea, severe vasospasms

3.22.) __DIURETICS__

		indications	☺ side effects
carb. anhydrase inhibitors	acetazolamide	- weak diuretic - rarely used	- metabolic acidosis [1]
loop diuretics	furosemide, ethacrynic acid	- acute pulmonary edema - hypercalcemia	- ototoxicity - hypokalemia - hyperuricemia
thiazides	chlorothiazide, hydrochlorothiazide, chlorthalidone	- hypertension - mild congestive heart failure - urinary calcium stones - diabetes insipidus	- hypokalemia - hypercalcemia - hyperglycemia - hyperuricemia
potassium sparing	spironolactone, (aldosterone antagonist) amiloride, triamterene	- usually combined with thiazides or loop diuretics - secondary hyperaldosteronism	- gynecomastia - menstrual irregularity
osmotic diuretics	mannitol	- acute renal failure - not useful in conditions a/w Na^+ retention	

[1] useful to prevent "mountain sickness" (respiratory alkalosis).

3.23.) ANTIANGINAL DRUGS

	key features
nitroglycerin	- low dose : dilates veins, reduces preload - high dose: also dilates arterioles, reflex tachycardia (angina may get worse)
isosorbide dinitrate	- orally active - less potent than nitroglycerin
nifedipine	- relaxes arterioles - best for Prinzmetal's angina (coronary artery spasm)
verapamil	- slows heart rate - effect partially overcome by reflex tachycardia

 *Nitroglycerin generates metHb (Fe^{3+}) which can
bind toxic cyanide - useful as an antidote!*

classic angina	myocardial infarction
- substernal pain	- substernal pain -> spreads to arms or jaw
- lasts < 10 minutes - relieved by rest and nitrates	- lasts > 30 minutes - not relieved by rest or nitrates

3.24.) <u>PLATELET AGGREGATION INHIBITORS</u>

 Prophylaxis of transient ischemic attacks (TIA).
Decreases mortality in postmyocardial patients.

	mechanism of action
aspirin	- inhibits cyclooxygenase (blocks thromboxane A_2 synthesis)
sulfinpyrazone	- inhibits degranulation (serotonin, ADP) - prolongs platelet survival
dipyridamole	- phosphodiesterase inhibitor - increases cAMP -> inhibits degranulation

---

- Prostacyclin -> increases platelet cAMP -> inhibits degranulation
- Thromboxane A_2 -> activates platelets (IP_3, DAG) -> degranulation

- Platelets release ADP and thromboxane A_2 -> activates other platelets

3.25.) ANTICOAGULANTS

	mechanism of action	antagonist
heparin	- enhances activity of antithrombin III	protamine sulfate
warfarin dicumarol	- antagonist of vit. K (II, VII, IX, X)	vitamin K
streptokinase	- derived from streptococci - activates plasminogen (plasmin then degrades fibrin)	aminocaproic acid
urokinase	- derived from human fetal renal cells - less antigenicity than streptokinase	
TPA	- "fibrin selective" [1]	

[1] activates only plasminogen already bound to fibrin

To monitor therapy with anticoagulants:
- **Warfarin:** prothrombin time (PT): extrinsic pathway
- **Heparin:** partial thromboplastin time (aPPT): intrinsic pathway

3.26.) <u>ANTIARRHYTHMIC DRUGS</u>

class 1	Na^+ channel blockers
class 2	β-blockers
class 3	K^+ channel blockers
class 4	Ca^{2+} channel blockers

class	drugs	APD	UV	indications
1A	quinidine, procainamide	↑	↓	- ectopic arrhythmias
1B	lidocaine, phenytoin	↓	↓	- acute ventricular flutter/fibrillation - digitalis induced arrhythmias
1C	flecainide encainide	∅	↓	- "broad spectrum" antiarrhythmic
2	propanolol			- atrial tachycardia - post MI (prophylactic)
3	bretylium amiodarone			- severe unresponsive ventricular arrhythmias
4	verapamil			- atrial tachycardia - atrial flutter

ADP: Action potential duration **UV:** Upstroke velocity

	SIDE-EFFECTS:
• **procainamide**:	reversible lupus erythematosus
• **phenytoin**:	gingiva hyperplasia
• **quinidine**:	potentiates digitoxin toxicity

3.27.) <u>INOTROPIC DRUGS</u>

increased strength of cardiac contractions -> increased stroke volume

		key features
glycosides	**digoxin, digitoxin**	- low therapeutic index!!! - digoxin: short, digitoxin: long action
β-agonists	**dobutamine, dopamine**	- increase cAMP - less tachycardia or peripheral side effects than isoproterenol or epinephrine
PDE inhibitors	**amrinone** **milrinone**	☹ thrombocytopenia ☺ does not affect platelets

Dopamine enhances renal blood flow and is particularly useful for treatment of shock.

GLYCOSIDE SIDE-EFFECTS:
- **extracardiac:** - nausea, abdominal pain
  - fatigue
  - confusion, disorientation
  - color misperception: yellow
- **cardiac:** - AV block, arrhythmias

<u>Toxicity of glycosides is enhanced by:</u>
- hypokalemia
- alkalosis
- hypoxia
- hypothyroidism

3.28.) <u>ASTHMA</u>

indication	mechanism of action	drug
mild, intermittent asthma	β_2-selective agonists	**metaproterenol, terbutaline, albuterol**
more severe asthma	phosphodiesterase inhibitor -> cAMP ↑	**theophylline**
prophylaxis	stabilize mast cells	**cromolyn**
severe, chronic asthma	anti-inflammatory	**corticosteroids** (inhaled)
status asthmaticus	anti-inflammatory	**corticosteroids I.V.**

<u>SIDE-EFFECTS:</u>
- **β_2-agonists**: - tremor
  - dizziness, palpitations
- **theophylline**: - arrhythmias, seizures
  (when overdosed!)

3.29.) <u>INSULINS</u>
for treatment of IDDM

		peak	duration
CZI	- "regular insulin"	30 min	120 min
semilente	- given subcutaneously - rapid onset	2-3 h	5-8 h
lente	- mix of semi and ultra	8-12 h	18-24 h
ultralente	- prolonged action	14-20 h	36 h
PZI	- CZI treated with protamine	24 h	36 h

Human insulin made by recombinant DNA techniques is increasingly popular.

<u>RISKS & SIDE-EFFECTS:</u>
- hypoglycemic reactions: sweating, anxiety, tremor, weakness
- allergy: beef > pork > human insulin
- fat atrophy at site of injection

A common schedule:
- mix CZI and NPH (lente)
- give twice daily (morning and evening)
- monitor glucose in morning and afternoon

3.30.) <u>SULFONYLUREAS</u>
for treatment of NIDDM

	duration of action
tolbutamide	8 h
glyburide, glipizide	20 h, most potent
chlorpropamide	48 h

Sulfonylureas are contraindicated in patients with liver or kidney failure: Accumulation will increase risk of hypoglycemia (especially with chlorpropamide)

 Sulfonylureas increase glucose sensitivity of β-cells.

3.31.) HYPERLIPIDEMIAS

LDL = Total Cholesterol - HDL - (Triglycerides / 5)

	elevated fraction	defect
Type I	chylomicrons *(triglycerides)*	lipoprotein lipase
Type IIA	LDL *(cholesterol)*	LDL receptor
Type IIB	LDL *(cholesterol)* VLDL *(triglycerides)*	mutant apoprotein ?
Type III	IDL *(triglycerides and cholesterol)*	mutant apoprotein E
Type IV	VLDL 1 *(triglycerides)*	overproduction of VLDL underutilization of VLDL

 Type IV (hypertriglyceridemia) does NOT increase the risk of coronary heart disease!

3.32.) <u>HYPERLIPIDEMIA DRUGS</u>

	mechanism of action / side-effects	indication
diet	- helps all types of hyperlipidemia - is the only option for type I	all
niacin	- inhibits lipolysis in fat cells - decreases free fatty acids (decreased VLDL synthesis) ☹ cutaneous flush	type IIB
clofibrate	- activates lipoprotein lipase (increases VLDL utilization) - inhibits cholesterol synthesis - enhances cholesterol excretion in bile ☹ forms gallstones	types III, IV
cholestyramine colestipol	- anion exchanger (binds cholesterol in gut) ☹ interferes with absorption of many drugs[1]	types IIA, IIB
lovastatin	- inhibits HMG-CoA reductase ☹ liver toxicity contraindicated during pregnancy	types IIA, IIB

[1] don't give at the same time of day!

3.33.) __PEPTIC ULCERS__

H₂ blockers	- **cimetidine**	☹ anti-androgenic action
	- **ranitidine**	- more potent, longer acting no anti-androgenic action
	- **famotidine**	- most potent
prostaglandins	- **misoprostol**	- analog of PGE
proton pump inhibitors	- **omeprazole**	- drug of choice !
anti muscarinic	- **pirenzepine**	- reduces acid secretion - less effect on motility - usually combined with others
antacids	- **Al (OH)₃**	☹ may cause constipation
	- **Mg (OH)₃**	☹ may cause diarrhea
mucosa protection	- **bismuth** - **sucralfate**	

> **Eradication of *H. pylori*:**
> metronidazole + tetracycline + bismuth

 Refractory ulcers -> suspect Zollinger-Ellison syndrome.
      (gastrinoma of pancreas or duodenum)

3.34.) ADRENERGIC DRUGS

		receptor action	main indications
α-blockers	- phenoxybenzamine	α1 , α2, irreversible	- autonomic hyperreflexia
	- phentolamine	α1 , α2, reversible	- hypertensive crisis
	- prazosin	α1	- hypertension
α-agonists	- phenylephrine	α1	- nasal decongestant
	- methoxamine	α1	- hypotension
	- clonidine	α2 , central action	- hypertension
β-blockers	- propanolol	β1 , β2	} hypertension
	- pindolol	β1 , β2 , intrinsic act.	migraine prophylaxis
	- metoprolol	β1	glaucoma
	- atenolol	β1	
	- labetalol	β , α	
β-agonists	- isoproterenol	β1 , β2	- AV block
	- metaproterenol, albuterol, terbutaline	β2	- bronchospasm
	- dobutamine	β1	- congestive heart failure
	- dopamine	D1 > β1	- shock
indirect -	- reserpine	depletes neuro-transmitter stores	- hypertension
	- guanethidine		- hypertension
indirect +	- ephedrine	prolongs neuro-transmitter action	- nasal decongestant
	- amphetamine		- narcolepsy, ADHD

159

3.35.) <u>CHOLINESTERASE INHIBITORS</u>

	use	key features
physostigmine	treatment of M.G.	☹ may cause CNS convulsions
neostigmine	treatment of M.G.	- does not enter CNS - better action on skeletal muscle
edrophonium	diagnosis of M.G.	- shortest duration of action
organophosphates	nerve gas insecticide	- irreversible (highly toxic)

M.G. = myasthenia gravis (autoantibodies against muscle ACh receptor)

DIAGNOSIS OF MYASTHENIA GRAVIS (TENSILON TEST):
- **Myasthenic crisis:** edrophonium improves muscle strength
- **Cholinergic crisis:** edrophonium further reduces muscle strength

---

Organophosphates directly inhibit ACh esterase and slowly form an irreversible complex with the esterase ("aging").
Pralidoxime prevents "aging" and releases active ACh esterase.

3.36.) <u>DIRECT CHOLINERGIC DRUGS</u>

	main indications	receptor action
bethanechol	- atonic bladder	muscarinic
pilocarpine [1]	- <u>acute</u> glaucoma	muscarinic
carbachol [1]	- glaucoma - not hydrolyzed by ACh-esterase	muscarinic and nicotinic

[1] produces miosis (small pupils)
   opens outflow (canal of Schlemm) -> reduces ocular pressure

Automatic bladder: *Spinal cord damage above sacral cord*
                    -> micturition reflex intact
               -> but loss of conscious control over reflex

Atonic bladder: *Caused by destruction of sensory nerves*
              Injury to sacral spinal cord -> loss of micturition reflex

           Spinal shock -> temporary loss of micturition reflex

3.37.) ANTIMUSCARINIC DRUGS

	use
atropine	- anti-spasmodic - mydriasis (large pupils) to facilitate ophthalmologic examination - antidote for organophosphate poisoning
scopolamine	- greater CNS action than atropine - for motion sickness

3.38.) ANTINICOTINIC DRUGS

	actions / use
tubocurarine	- blocks nicotinic ACh receptor - muscle relaxant (surgery) ☹ histamine release -> bronchospasm hypotension
pancuronium	☺ less histamine release than tubocurarine
succinyl choline	- depolarizing - very short duration of action ☹ post-op muscle pain and stiffness risk of malignant hyperthermia [1]

[1] Ca^{2+} release from SR -> muscles generate heat -> life threatening!

> ***Be careful with drugs that***
> ***enhance neuromuscular block:***
> - *halothane*
> - *aminoglycosides*
> - *Ca^{2+} channel blockers*

3.39.) SEX-HORMONES

SIDE-EFFECTS:

ESTROGENS	PROGESTERONES
☹ nausea vomiting breast tenderness skin pigmentation hypertension breakthrough bleeding	☹ weight gain depression hirsutism

USES:

estrogen	- "**morning after pill**"
progesterone	- "**mini pill**" - habitual abortion - endometriosis
combination	- oral contraceptive - hormone replacement

Risks of Oral Contraceptives:
- thromboembolia
- benign adenoma of the liver
- vaginal cancer in daughters of mothers who received DES

- **but not** : breast cancer or endometrial cancer
  (provided estrogen is combined with progesterone!)

3.40.) HALLUCINOGENS

	key features
LSD	- acts on 5-HT$_1$ and 5-HT$_2$ receptors
	- activates sympathetic system -> arousal, tachycardia, sweating
	- brilliant color hallucinations (these are blockable by neuroleptics)
	- may trigger schizophreniform psychosis
	- flashbacks
THC (marihuana)	- enhanced sensory activity
	- impaired mental activity, sleepiness
	- altered sense of time and self
	- impaired short term memory
	- red conjunctivas
phencyclidine ("angel dust")	- reuptake inhibitor
	- mood elevation, sense of intoxication
	- bizarre and aggressive behavior

 Flashback: *Recurrence of drug effect without the drug.*

3.41.) OPIOIDS

Endorphins (endogenous opioid peptides):

	receptor	effect
met-enkephalin	mu	- euphoria, dependence - analgesia - respiratory depression
leu-enkephalin	delta	- mood changes
dynorphin	kappa	- analgesia, miosis, sedation

Morphine (like met-enkephalin) acts on mu receptors.

Synthetic opioids:

	key features
naloxone	- μ, κ, σ antagonist - reverses morphine overdose
pentazocine	- κ, σ agonist / δ, μ antagonist - less effective for severe pain than morphine - less potential for dependence
codeine	- weak analgesic ("as strong as aspirin") - good antitussive - low abuse potential
propoxyphene	- **dextro** : analgesic - **levo** : antitussive
fentanyl	- 80x analgesic potency of morphine
methadone	- longer duration of action than morphine - used for controlled withdrawal

3.42.) <u>ANTIDEPRESSANTS</u>

	mechanism of action	key features
Tricyclic antidepressants amitriptyline amoxapine desipramine etc.	- block neurotransmitter uptake (NE, serotonin, dopamine) - block receptors (m, α, serotonin, histamine)	- slow onset of action - inconsistent bioavailability ☹ **anticholinergic:** - blurred vision, dry mouth - constipation - urinary retention
imipramine		- for enuresis
"Next Generation" fluoxetine trazodone	- selectively block uptake of serotonin	☺ few anticholinergic effects
MAO inhibitors	- increases amount of transmitter stored	- "second choice" - have stimulant properties - caveat : tyramine

Tyramine (cheese, beer, red wine) normally is inactivated by MAO in gut.
When it gets into the circulation -> hypertensive crisis!

166

3.43.) <u>LITHIUM</u>
Therapeutic range: 0.5-1 mEq/L

key features	☹ extremely low therapeutic index - excreted by kidneys
indications	- to treat manic episodes - to stabilize mood (prevents both manic and depressive episodes)
"normal" side-effects	- mild nausea - thirst
early intoxication 1.5 - 2 mEq/L	- abdominal pain, vomiting - hand tremor - ataxia, nystagmus - slurred speech
severe intoxication > 2 mEq/L	- persistent vomiting - blurred vision - hyperactive tendon reflexes - convulsions, coma, death

3.44.) <u>CNS STIMULANTS</u>

	key features
methylxanthines caffeine, theophylline	- low dose : increased alertness - high dose : anxiety, tremors - smooth muscle relaxation - weak diuretic - enhanced HCl secretion in stomach
nicotine	- low dose : ganglion stimulating, BP↑ - high dose: ganglion blockade, BP↓
cocaine	- reuptake inhibitor - local anesthetic and vasoconstrictor - euphoria, hallucinations delusions, paranoia - cardiac arrhythmias
amphetamines	- release of stored catecholamines - effects like cocaine - euphoria lasts longer than cocaine - no tolerance to CNS toxicity

Dextroamphetamine: *- strong appetite suppressant*
                              - euphoria, risk of dependence
                              - not recommended for weight loss!

<u>Attention-Deficit-Hyperactivity-Disorder:</u>
Children with ADHD have a "paradoxical" reaction
to amphetamines: It calms them down!

3.45.) <u>ANXIOLYTIC DRUGS</u>

		key features
benzodiazepines	**diazepam**	- long acting - for status epilepticus
	chlordiazepoxide	- long acting - for alcohol withdrawal
	lorazepam, triazolam	- rapid elimination (short half life) -> ☹ severe withdrawal symptoms
others	**buspirone**	- acts on 5-HT$_{1A}$ receptors - slow onset of action - little sedation - little dependence

 Abrupt withdrawal may cause delirium and seizures!

3.46.) <u>HYPNOTIC DRUGS</u>

		key features
barbiturates	**phenobarbital**	- long acting, for seizure disorder
	thiopental	- short acting, for anesthesia
others	**chloral hydrate**	- recommended for children ☹ causes epigastric pain
	meprobamate	- less sedation, better anxiolytic

3.47.) <u>ANTIHISTAMINES</u>

	key features
diphenhydramine	<u>indications:</u> - allergic rhinitis - urticaria - not effective in asthma ☹ sedation
carbinoxamine	☺ less drowsiness than diphenhydramine
trimeprazine (phenothiazine)	- long half life - good antipruritic
terfenadine, **astemizole**	- non-sedating antihistamines

<u>For motion sickness and nausea:</u>
- diphenhydramine (antihistamine)
- meclizine (antihistamine)
- scopolamine (phenothiazine)

3.48.) ANESTHETICS

MAC :	$N_2O > ether > enflurane > halothane$
onset :	$N_2O > enflurane > halothane > ether$
	fastest........................slowest

Inhalation:

	key features

halothane	- lacks analgesic potency
	 ☹ hepatotoxic for adults
	     cardiac arrhythmias
	     malignant hyperthermia

enflurane	- excreted by kidney rather than liver
isoflurane	- does not induce arrhythmias - lower toxicity
N_2O	- not potent - does not depress respiration - safe

I.V.:

thiopental	- ultrashort barbiturate - not analgesic
ketamine	- dissociative anesthesia (patient appears awake but is unaware of pain) ☹ postoperative hallucinations

---

Examples:
- **balanced anesthesia** : thiopental + fentanyl + tubocurarine + N_2O
- **neurolept anesthesia** : droperidol + fentanyl + N_2O

3.49.) PARKINSON'S DISEASE

dopaminergic	**levodopa** (**plus carbidopa**	- CNS permeable dopamine
		- to inhibit peripheral decarboxylase)
		
		☹ nausea, vomiting
		   dyskinesia
		   psychic disturbances

	bromocriptine	- direct dopamine agonist
	deprenyl	- inhibits MAO-B (dopamine selective)
	amantadine	- enhances dopamine metabolism

anticholinergic	**benztropine**
	biperiden
		☹ dry mouth
		   mydriasis
		   tachycardia
		   constipation
		   urinary retention

Early disease:
- If symptoms are mild, no drugs may be necessary
- Otherwise start with anticholinergics or amantadine

Fully developed disease:
- Levodopa plus Carbidopa

Late stage:
- "wearing off" of drug effect
- "on-off" phenomenon
- may need to reduce levodopa if dyskinesias develop
- may need to combine several drugs

3.50.) NEUROLEPTICS

		key features
phenothiazines	**chlorpromazine**	☹ anticholinergic side effects arrhythmias rarely used
	fluphenazine	- long acting - for outpatients
butyrophenones	**haloperidol**	☹ extrapyramidal side effects fewer anticholinergic side effects
	droperidol	- for neurolept anesthesia
other	**clozapine**	☹ bone marrow suppression fewer extrapyramidal side effects

---

☹ **DYSKINESIAS CAUSED BY NEUROLEPTICS:**
- **Acute dystonia occurs within hours of administration**
  torticollis, jaw dislocation, tongue protrusion
  usually disappears (tolerance)

- **Parkinsonism occurs within weeks to months of treatment**
  muscle stiffness, cogwheel rigidity, shuffling, drooling
  usually disappears (tolerance)

- **Tardive dyskinesia occurs after many months of treatment**
  choreoathetosis, tongue protrusion, lateral movements of jaw
  may be irreversible!

3.51.) <u>ANTIEPILEPTIC DRUGS</u>

disorder	drug of choice
partial focal	phenytoin, carbamazepine
grand mal	phenytoin, carbamazepine
petit mal	ethosuximide
myoclonic	valproic acid, clonazepam
febrile seizures (children)	phenobarbital
status epilepticus [1]	diazepam, phenytoin I.V.

[1] *Medical emergency! Keep airways open!*

3.52.) ANTIEMETIC DRUGS

underlying cause	drug of choice
motion sickness	scopolamine, diphenhydramine
vertigo	meclizine
chemotherapy	metoclopramide
radiation therapy	domperidone

3.53.) LAXATIVES

bulk forming [1] (stool softeners)	- fibers (fruit, vegetable) - methyl cellulose - psyllium seeds
irritants (increased intestinal motility)	- senna - castor oil
nonabsorbable salines [1] (increased osmotic pressure)	- magnesium salts
lubricants (to protect hemorrhoids)	- mineral oil

[1] take with plenty of water

Abuse of laxatives -> *intestinal potassium loss* -> *hypokalemia* -> *decreased intestinal motility* -> *increased "need" for laxatives*

BIOCHEMISTRY

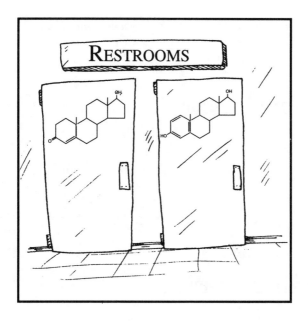

RESTROOMS

4.1.) <u>ENZYME KINETICS</u>

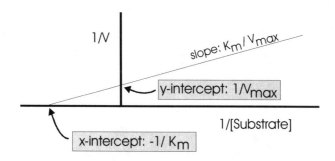

V_{max}: *Maximal rate of reaction when enzyme is saturated with substrate.*

K_m: *Substrate concentration at which reaction rate is half of its maximal value.*
High K_m = low affinity
Low K_m = high affinity

<u>COMPETITIVE INHIBITOR:</u>

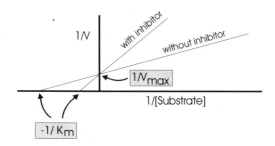

<u>NONCOMPETITIVE INHIBITOR:</u>

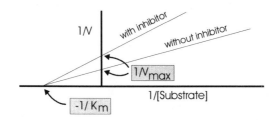

4.2.) <u>AMINO ACIDS</u>

acidic	aspartate, glutamate
basic	histidine, lysine, arginine
essential	valine, leucin, isoleucine tryptophan, phenylalanine, methionine lysine, arginine histidine, threonine
strictly ketogenic	leucine, lysine
keto- and glucogenic	isoleucine, threonine tryptophan, phenylalanine

Glucogenic: if carbon skeleton can be converted to glucose.
Ketogenic: if carbon skeleton can be converted to acetyl CoA.

trypsin cleaves at	$^+NH_3$ - ⬚ Arg or Lys - ⬚ any - COO^-
chymotrypsin cleaves at	$^+NH_3$ - ⬚ Phe, Tyr, Trp or Leu - ⬚ any - COO^-

4.3.) AMINO ACID PRECURSORS

Many important molecules are made from amino acids:

	products:
tyrosine	- dopa, dopamine - norepinephrine, epinephrine - T_3, T_4 (thyroxin) - melanin
tryptophan	- 5-HT (serotonin) - melatonin - niacin
glutamate	- GABA
glycine	- porphyrin, heme - creatine (glycine plus + arginine)
histidine	- histamine

4.4.) <u>AMINO ACID DISORDERS</u>

	enzyme	signs & symptoms
albinism	tyrosinase	- unpigmented skin, eyes
phenylketonuria	phenylalanine hydroxylase	- mental retardation - hypopigmentation - musty odor
alkaptonuria	homogentisate oxidase	- arthritis (ochronosis) - urine darkens
maple syrup	branched chain dehydrogenase	- hyperreflexia - sweet odor urine
homocystinuria	cystathionine synthetase	- mental retardation - lens dislocation
cystinuria	dibasic amino acid transporter [1]	- urinary cystine stones
Hartnup disease	neutral amino acid transporter [1]	- tryptophan deficiency ↓ niacin deficiency ↓ pellagra

[1] *Same transporters are also defective in intestinal epithelium -> patients do not absorb these amino acids from digestive products in the intestinal lumen.*

<u>Pellagra</u> (Hartnup disease or dietary niacin deficiency):
3 "D"s: • dermatitis   • dementia   • diarrhea

4.5.) ENZYME DEFECTS

ALBINISM:

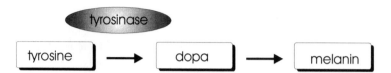

Albinism is due to defective tyrosinase in melanocytes. Nerve cell tyrosinase is intact (patients can still make epinephrine and norepinephrine).

PHENYLKETONURIA:

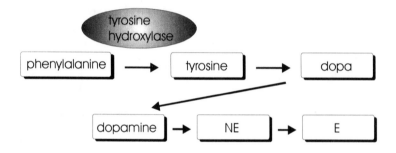

Tyrosine become an essential amino acid in patients with phenylketonuria.

ALKAPTONURIA:

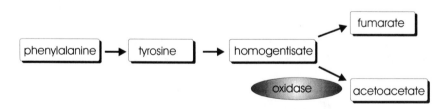

MAPLE SYRUP DISEASE:

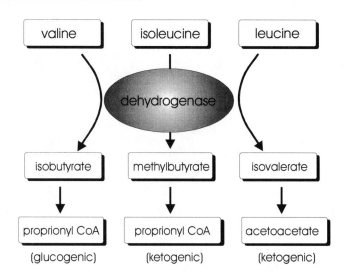

valine	isoleucine	leucine

dehydrogenase

isobutyrate	methylbutyrate	isovalerate

proprionyl CoA	proprionyl CoA	acetoacetate
(glucogenic)	(ketogenic)	(ketogenic)

HOMOCYSTINURIA:

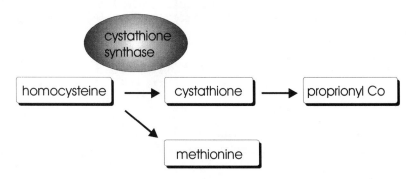

cystathione synthase

homocysteine → cystathione → proprionyl Co

methionine

homocysteine + homocysteine -> homocystine

4.6.) <u>HEXOSES</u>

<u>EPIMERS OF GLUCOSE:</u>

αD-glucose	mannose	galactose
β CHO α	CHO	CHO
2- OH	OH - 2	2- OH
OH - 3	OH - 3	OH - 3
4-OH	4-OH	OH - 4
L 5-OH D	5-OH	5-OH
CH_2OH	CH_2OH	CH_2OH

pyranose	- ring with <u>5 carbons + 1 oxygen</u> (example: glucose)
furanose	- ring with <u>4 carbons + 1 oxygen</u> (example: fructose)
anomeric carbon	- C atom that has <u>4 different ligands</u> (for sugars this refers to the C1 in ring form)
epimers	- isomers that differ in only <u>one</u> carbon (example: glucose and galactose)
enantiomers	- mirror image (i.e. flipped at all anomeric C atoms)
reducing sugars	- oxygen on C1 atom is available for redox reaction - glucose, galactose and fructose are reducing sugars - sucrose is a non-reducing sugar

4.7.) <u>HEXOSE KINASES</u>

	hexokinase	glucokinase
tissues	many	liver, β-cells
substrate specificity	hexoses	same !
affinity	high	low
V_{max} ("capacity")	low	high
inhibited by glucose-6-phosphate	yes	no

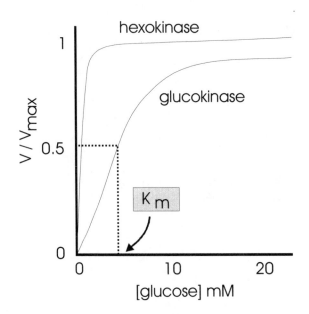

4.8.) <u>SACCHARIDES</u>

<u>DISACCHARIDES</u>:

	composition	bond
maltose	glucose + glucose	$\alpha 1 - 4$
lactose	galactose + glucose	$\beta 1 - 4$
sucrose	glucose + fructose	$\alpha 1 - \beta 2$

<u>POLYSACCHARIDES</u>:

	composition	bonds
glycogen, starch	many glucoses	$\alpha 1 - 4$ (chains) $\alpha 1 - 6$ (branch points)
cellulose	many glucoses	$\beta 1 - 4$

 The $\beta 1$- 4 bond cannot be hydrolyzed by humans.
(Cellulose is indigestible.)

4.9.) <u>SACCHARIDE DISORDERS</u>

	enzyme defect	signs & symptoms
fructosuria	fructokinase	- benign - asymptomatic
fructose intolerance	aldolase B	- hypoglycemia - liver failure
galactosemia	uridyltransferase	- cataracts - mental retardation
lactose intolerance	lactase (usually acquired)	- diarrhea

 Diarrhea of any cause can result in temporary lactase deficiency.
(Don't drink milk if you have diarrhea!)

4.10.) <u>ENZYME DEFECTS</u>

<u>FRUCTOSE INTOLERANCE:</u>

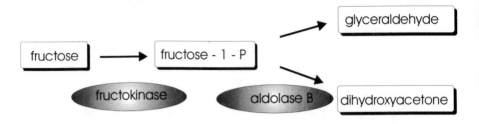

Fructosuria *(defective fructokinase): Fructose is harmless.*

Fructose intolerance *(defective aldolase): Fructose-1-P accumulates in liver and inhibits glycogenolysis and gluconeogenesis -> severe hypoglycemia.*

<u>GALACTOSEMIA:</u>

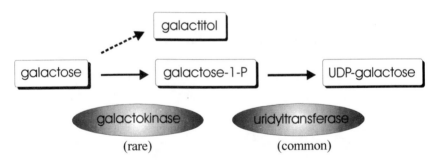

Many States in the US require newborn screening for this disease because failure to treat results in early mental retardation.

4.11.) <u>GLYCOGEN STORAGE DISEASES</u>

	enzyme defect	organs affected
Type I Von Gierke	glucose-6-phosphatase	- liver and kidneys enlarged - fasting hypoglycemia - acidosis - failure to thrive
Type II Pompe	α-glucosidase (lysosomes)	- affects all organs - muscle hypotonia - cardiac failure - death before age 2
Type V McArdle	skeletal muscle phosphorylase	- exercise: muscle pain/cramps - progressive muscle weakness

Skeletal muscle cells don't have glucose-6-phosphatase (unlike the liver, muscle cells do not release glucose into the circulation).

4.12.) <u>ENZYME DEFECTS</u>

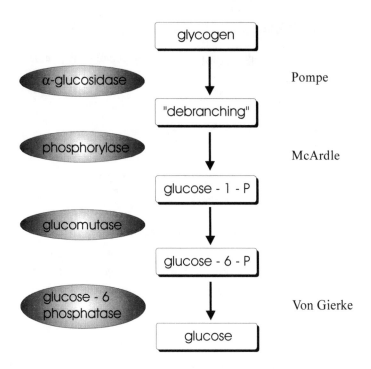

	glycogen	
α-glucosidase	↓	Pompe
	"debranching"	
phosphorylase	↓	McArdle
	glucose - 1 - P	
glucomutase	↓	
	glucose - 6 - P	
glucose - 6 phosphatase	↓	Von Gierke
	glucose	

4.13.) GLYCOSAMINOGLYCANS

> Long, unbranched polysaccharides composed of repeating disaccharides.
> One of the disaccharides is a hexosamine (often N-acetyl-glucosamine).

Common glycosaminoglycans (=mucopolysaccharides):
- hyaluronic acid
- heparin
- keratan sulfate
- chondroitin sulfate
- dermatan sulfate

SOME MUCOPOLYSACCHARIDOSES:

	enzyme defect	signs & symptoms
Hurler	α-L Iduronidase [2]	- cornea clouding - mental retardation
Scheie	α-L Iduronidase [2]	- cornea clouding - normal intelligence
Hunter	Iduronate sulfatase	- no clouding - mental retardation

[2] *these are different mutations!*

PROTEOGLYCANS:

- Proteoglycans have a protein core to which numerous side chains of glycosaminoglycans attach.
- Major functions: Lubricants, extracellular matrix, molecular "sieve".

4.14.) <u>FATTY ACIDS</u>

<u>SATURATED:</u>

	structure	features
palmitic acid	16:0	- product of human fatty acid synthesis
stearic acid	18:0	

<u>MONOUNSATURATED:</u>

palmitoleic acid	16:1(9)	
oleic acid	18:1(9)	

<u>POLYUNSATURATED:</u>

linoleic acid **linolenic acid**	18:2(9,12) 18:3(9,12,15)	- plant oils
arachidonic acid	20:4(5,8,11,14)	- precursor of prostaglandins

Example: 18:1(9): *18 carbons, 1 double bond at position 9*

- *Peripheral atherosclerosis correlates with saturated fat intake.*
- *Margarine (hydrogenated vegetable oils = <u>trans</u> fatty acids)*
  is similarly harmful.

4.15.) <u>BILE ACIDS</u>

	bile acids	features
primary	- cholic acid - chenodeoxycholic acid	derived from cholesterol
secondary	- deoxycholic acid - lithocholic acid	produced from primary conjugated bile salts by intestinal bacteria less soluble -> excreted

conjugate	- glycocholic acid
	  (cholic acid + glycine)
	
	- taurocholic acid
	  (cholic acid + taurine)
	
	etc...
		ionized at physiologic pH
		
		form micelles with dietary fats

 >95% of bile salts are reabsorbed in the ileum.
("Enterohepatic circulation")

4.16.) <u>PHOSPHOLIPIDS</u>

<u>TRIGLYCERIDES</u>　　　　<u>GLYCERO-PHOSPHOLIPIDS</u>

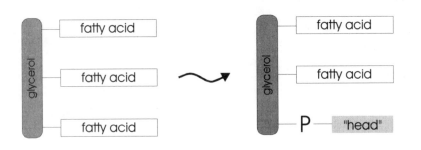

<u>CERAMIDE</u>　　　　<u>SPHINGO-PHOSPHOLIPIDS</u>

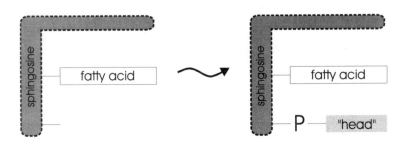

<u>CEREBROSIDES</u>　　　　<u>GANGLIOSIDES</u>

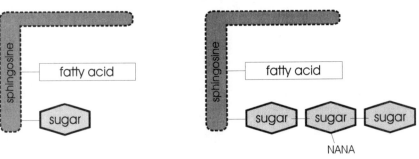

194

GLYCERO-PHOSPHOLIPIDS:
(spontaneously form lipid bilayers -> cell membranes)

phosphatidyl choline (= lecithin)	phosphatidic acid + choline
phosphatidyl ethanolamine	phosphatidic acid + ethanolamine
phosphatidyl serine	phosphatidic acid + serine
phosphatidyl inositol	phosphatidic acid + inositol
cardiolipin	2x phosphatidic acid + glycerine

= "head"

4.17.) SPHINGOLIPIDS

SPHINGO-PHOSPHOLIPIDS:

ceramide	sphingosine + fatty acid
sphingomyelin	ceramide + choline

SPHINGO-GLYCOLIPIDS:

cerebroside	ceramide + mono saccharide
globoside	ceramide + oligosaccharide
ganglioside	ceramide + oligosaccharide + NANA

4.18.) SPHINGOLIPIDOSES

		accumulate/enzyme	signs & symptoms
Niemann-Pick	A	sphingomyelin/ sphingomyelinase	- liver and spleen enlargement - foamy cells
Gaucher	A	glucocerebrosides/ β-glucosidase	- liver and spleen enlargement - osteoporosis - Ashkenazi Jews
Krabbe	A	galactocerebrosides/ β-galactosidase	- blindness, deafness - convulsions - globoid cells
metachromatic leukodystrophy	A	sulfatides/ arylsulfatase	- progressive paralysis
Fabry	X	globosides/ α-galactosidase	- reddish-purple skin rash - kidney/heart failure - angiokeratoma
Tay-Sachs	A	gangliosides/ hexosaminidase	- blindness - cherry red macula - Ashkenazi Jews

A: Autosomal recessive
X: X-linked recessive

4.19.) __ENZYME DEFECTS__

GALACTOSE:

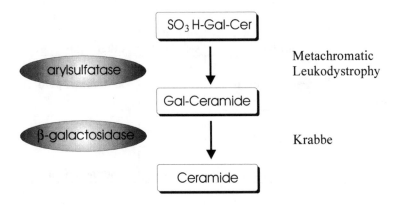

SO$_3$H-Gal-Cer

arylsulfatase   Metachromatic
                                 Leukodystrophy

Gal-Ceramide

β-galactosidase   Krabbe

Ceramide

GLUCOSE:

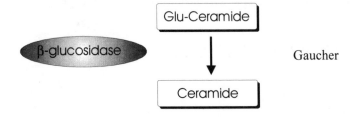

Glu-Ceramide

β-glucosidase   Gaucher

Ceramide

4.20.) PORPHYRIAS

Defects in heme biosynthesis

	accumulate	photo-sensitivity	other signs
acute intermittent	porphobilinogen [1]	no	**abdominal pain**
cutanea tarda	uroporphyrinogen	**yes**	
coproporphyria	coproporphyrinogen	**yes**	**abdominal pain**
lead poisoning	δ-ALA protoporphyrin	no	**anemia** *- microcytic, hypochrome - basophil stippling*

[1] precipitated by dieting, steroids, sulfonamides and many other drugs.

MECHANISM OF PHOTOSENSITIVITY:

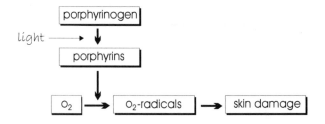

198

4.21.) **ENZYME DEFECTS**

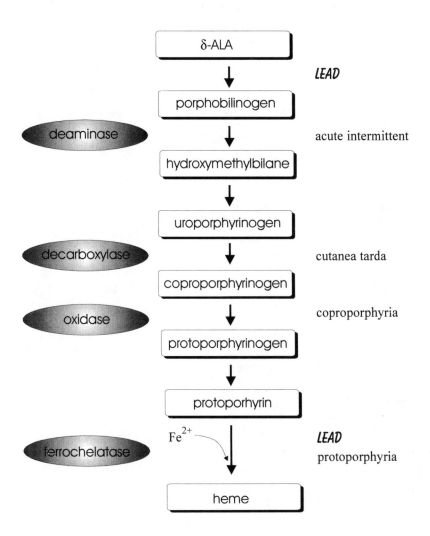

4.22.) PREFERRED FUELS

After a prolonged fast, metabolism adapts to preserve amino acids:

	normal	prolonged fast
brain	- glucose	- ketone bodies - glucose
muscle	- **rest**: fatty acids - **exercise**: glucose	- fatty acids
heart ("ready for anything")	- fatty acids - ketone bodies - lactate - glucose	- fatty acids - ketone bodies - lactate - glucose
erythrocytes	- glucose	- glucose

 The heart is completely aerobic. In contrast, skeletal muscles can function anaerobically for some time.

FASTING:
- The brain and red blood cells always need glucose.
- The liver maintains glucose levels by a) Glycogenolysis
  b) Gluconeogenesis

- Substrates for liver gluconeogenesis: Muscle, RBCs: -> lactate
  Fat cells: triglycerides -> glycerol

- Production of ketones by liver: Triglycerides -> fatty acids -> ketones

4.23.) <u>VITAMINS</u>

A	- part of rhodopsin	- night blindness (retinal) - growth retardation (retinoic acid)
D	- GI tract: Ca^{2+} absorption - bone : supports PTH	- rickets, osteomalacia
E	- antioxidant	- ataxia
K	- carboxylation of glutamate	- bleeding disorder (II, VII, IX, X)
C	- hydroxylation of proline and lysine	- scurvy
B1 (thiamin)	- decarboxylations	- beriberi
B2 (riboflavin)	- flavins (FMN etc.)	- glossitis, cheilosis
B6 (pyridoxine)	- transaminations - deaminations	- anemia (microcytic) - neuropathy
B12	- methionine synthesis - odd carbon fatty acid degradation	- anemia (macrocytic) - neuropathy - *D. Latum* !
niacin	- NAD^+, NADPH	- pellagra (diarrhea, dementia, dermatitis)
pantothenate	- CoA	- headache, nausea
biotin	- carboxylations	- seborrheic dermatitis - nervous disorders - *avidin (raw egg white) binds biotin*
folic acid	- one carbon metabolism	- anemia (macrocytic) - glossitis, colitis

4.24.) <u>ATP EQUIVALENTS</u>

	yield	explanation
FADH$_2$	2	
NADH	3	
acetyl CoA	12	acetyl CoA -> 2 CO_2 3 NADH + FADH$_2$ + GTP
pyruvate	15	pyruvate -> acetyl CoA + NADH
glycolysis (anaerobe)	2	glucose -> lactate 4 ATP minus 2 ATP [1]
glycolysis (aerobe)	8	glucose -> pyruvate (4 ATP minus 2 ATP) + 2 NADH
glucose (complete oxidation)	38	glucose -> 6 CO_2 8 + 2x15 (pyruvate)
fatty acid (e.g. 16:0)	129	
gluconeogenesis (from pyruvate)	-12	
urea synthesis	-4	

[1] 2 ATP required for hexokinase and fructokinase reactions

Glycerophosphate shuttle (yields 2 ATP per NADH)
Reducing equivalents are transferred from cytosolic NADH to mitochondrial FADH$_2$.

Malate shuttle (yields 3 ATP per NADH)
Reducing equivalents are transferred from cytosolic NADH to mitochondrial NADH.

4.25.) KEY ENZYMES - SUGARS

	enzyme	–	+	phosphorylation
glycolysis	phosphofructokinase 1	ATP citrate	AMP fructose 2,6 -dp	
	phosphofructokinase 2			inhibits
gluconeogenesis	fructosediphosphatase 1	AMP fructose 2,6 -dp	ATP citrate	
	fructosediphosphatase 2			activates
glycogenolysis	glycogenphosphorylase			activates
glycogen synthesis	glycogen synthetase			inhibits
pentose phosphate shunt	glucose-6-phosphate dehydrogenase	NADPH		

– : allosteric inhibitor
+: allosteric activator

203

4.26.) KEY ENZYMES - FATS

	enzyme	-	+	phosphorylation
lipolysis	carnitine acyltransferase	malonyl CoA		
fat mobilization	hormone sensitive lipase			activates
lipid synthesis	acetyl-CoA carboxylase		citrate	inhibits
cholesterol synthesis	HMG CoA reductase		cholesterol	inhibits

- : allosteric inhibitor
+: allosteric activator

4.27.) KEY ENZYMES - OTHERS

	enzyme	—	phosphorylation
ketone body synthesis	HMG CoA synthase		
purine synthesis	amidotransferase	AMP GMP IMP	
citric acid cycle	pyruvate dehydrogenase		inhibits Acetyl CoA ATP NADH

— : allosteric inhibitor

205

4.28.) <u>STEROIDS</u>

class	example	number of C-atoms
sterols	cholesterol	27
bile acids	glycocholate taurocholate	24
glucocorticoids	cortisol	21
mineralocorticoids	aldosterone	21
gestagens	progesterone	21
androgens	testosterone * androstenedione DHEAS	19
estrogens	estradiol * estriol	18

* most potent

<u>17-ketosteroids</u> **(dehydroandrosterone and androstenedione):**
Increased: 11-hydroxylase deficiency
                     21-hydroxylase deficiency
                     Cushing's syndrome
                     androgen producing adrenal or gonadal tumors

<u>17-hydroxysteroids</u> **(cortisol metabolites):**
Increased: 11-hydroxylase deficiency
                     Cushing's syndrome

4.29.) <u>ADRENAL GLAND</u>

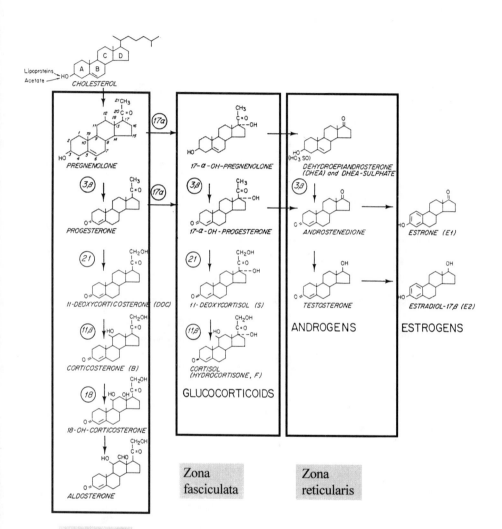

Zona glomerulosa

Zona fasciculata

Zona reticularis

4.30.) __TESTIS (Leydig Cells)__

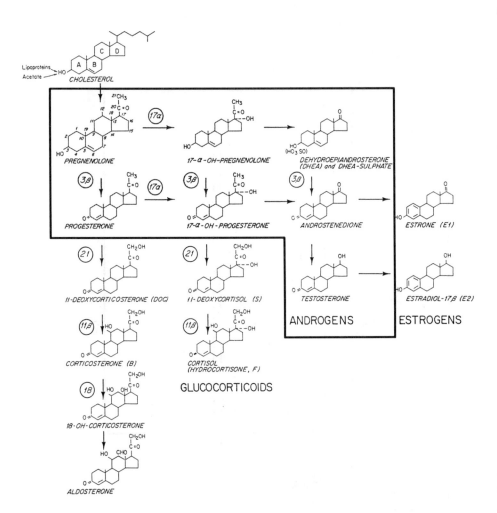

ANDROGENS ESTROGENS

GLUCOCORTICOIDS

4.31.) <u>PERIPHERAL METABOLISM</u>

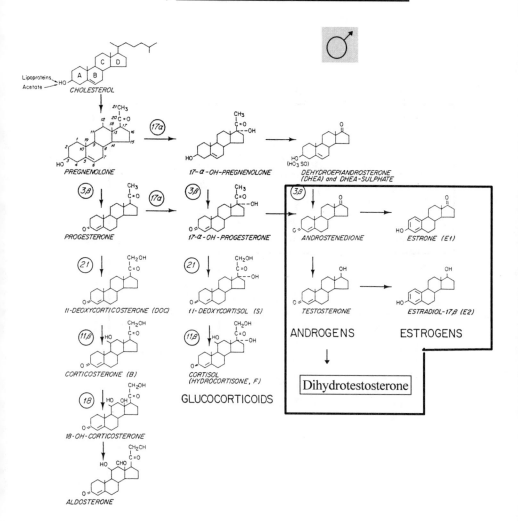

209

4.32.) <u>OVARY (Theca Cells)</u>

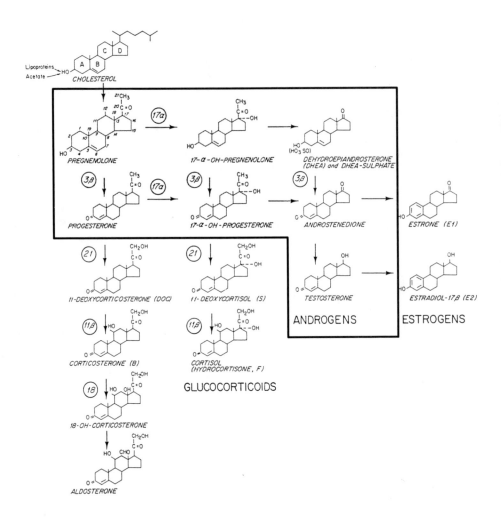

4.33.) <u>OVARY (Granulosa Cells)</u>

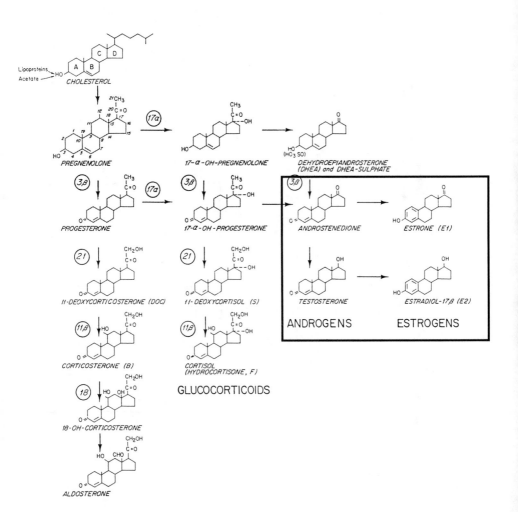

211

4.34.) **PERIPHERAL METABOLISM**

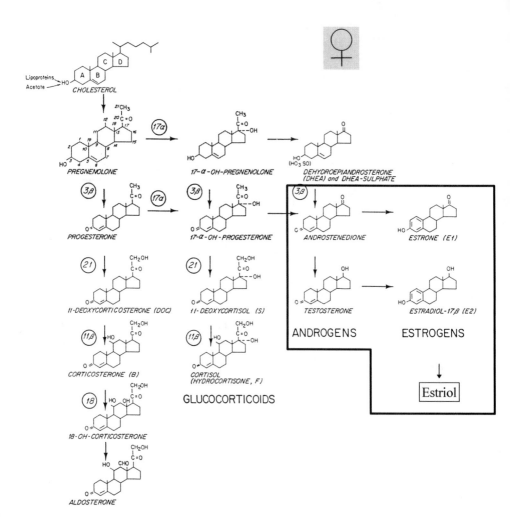

4.35.) <u>CORPUS LUTEUM</u>

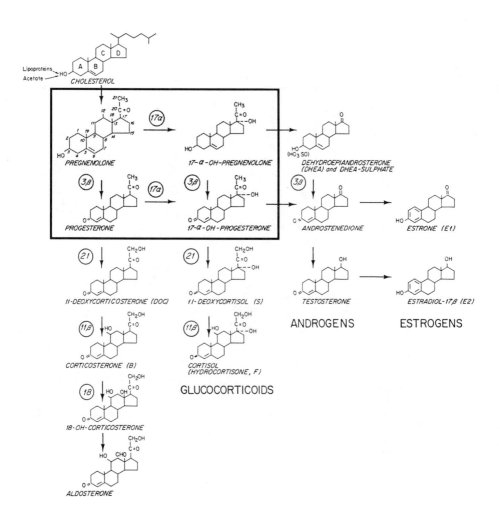

213

4.36.) 17-α-HYDROXYLASE DEFICIENCY

Male :	ambiguous genitalia
Female :	primary amenorrhea at puberty

4.37.) 21-α-HYDROXYLASE DEFICIENCY

most common defect of
corticoid synthesis (95%)

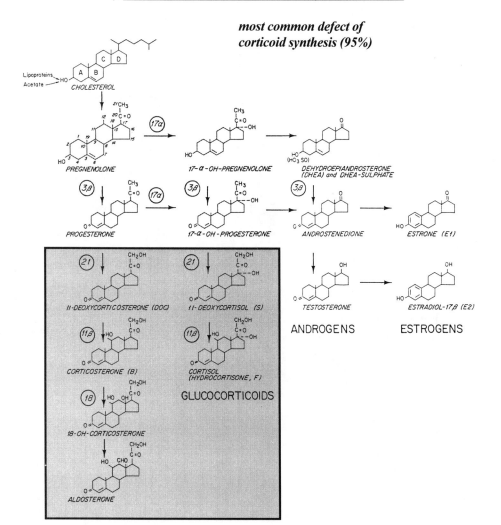

Male :	precocious puberty (DHEA↑)	
Female :	ambiguous genitalia (DHEA↑)	
Salt wasting:	50-60% of patients (lack of aldosterone)	

4.38.) 11-β-HYDROXYLASE

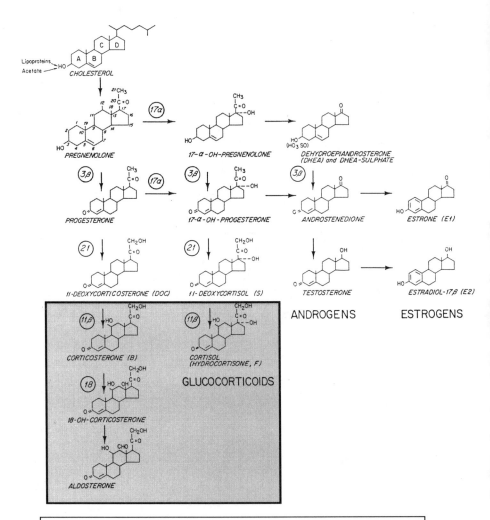

Male :	precocious puberty (androgens↑)	
Female :	ambiguous genitalia (androgens↑)	
Salt retention:	hypertension, hypokalemia	
	(deoxycorticosterone has mineralocorticoid action)	

4.39.) ENDOCRINE CONTROL OF METABOLISM

	fat	sugar	proteins
insulin	(A) synthesis	(A) uptake (M,F) glycolysis (L,M) glycogen synthesis (L,M)	(A) synthesis
glucagon	(C) lysis	(C) gluconeogenesis (L) glycogenolysis (L)	(C) increases uptake of AA in liver for gluconeogenesis
growth hormone	(C) lysis	(C) gluconeogenesis (L)	(A) synthesis
cortisol	(C) lysis redistribution	(A) inhibits uptake (M,F) gluconeogenesis (L) glycogen synthesis (L)	(C) degradation
epinephrine	(C) lysis	(C) increases uptake (M) glycolysis (M) gluconeogenesis (L) glycogenolysis (L,M)	-

(A) anabolic   (C) catabolic   M: Muscle   L: Liver   F: Fat

217

4.40.) <u>NUCLEOTIDES</u>

base	nucleoside	nucleotide
PURINES:		
adenine	adenosine	adenylate (AMP)
guanine	guanosine	guanylate (GMP)
PYRIMIDINES:		
uracil	uridine	uridylate (UMP)
cytosine	cytidine	cytidylate (CMP)
thymine	deoxythymidine	deoxythymidylate (dTMP)

<u>**Thymidine:**</u>　　　　　　　<u>**AZT:**</u>

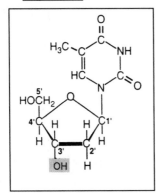　　　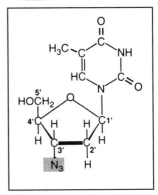

*AZT (Zidovudine) can be incorporated into DNA by viral
reverse transcriptase. Lack of the 3'-OH group then
inhibits further elongation of DNA.*

*Mammalian polymerase is less likely to "mistake" AZT for
thymidine.*

4.41.) <u>PURINES</u>

De novo synthesis (in liver from amino acid precursors):

1.) | phosphoribosyl pyrophosphate | → | IMP |

2.) | IMP | → | AMP or GMP | → | ADP or GDP |

Salvage of purine bases (react with PPRP to form nucleotides):

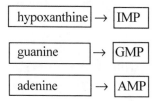

| hypoxanthine | → | IMP |

| guanine | → | GMP |

| adenine | → | AMP |

Lesch-Nyhan: *Defective phosphoribosyl transferase: Purine bases cannot be salvaged and are all degraded to uric acid -> gout, severe neurological signs.*

Degradation of purine bases (in liver):

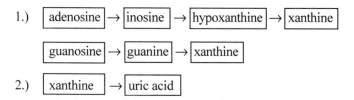

1.) | adenosine | → | inosine | → | hypoxanthine | → | xanthine |

| guanosine | → | guanine | → | xanthine |

2.) | xanthine | → | uric acid |

Allopurinol *inhibits conversion of xanthine to uric acid and is used for treatment of gout.*

4.42.) <u>PYRIMIDINES</u>

<u>De novo synthesis</u> (in liver):

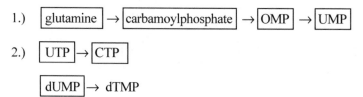

1.) | glutamine | → | carbamoylphosphate | → | OMP | → | UMP |

2.) | UTP | → | CTP |

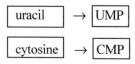

| dUMP | → dTMP

5-Fluorouracil *(anti cancer drug) is converted by the same enzymes to 5-FdUMP which is a potent inhibitor of thymidine synthesis.*

<u>Salvage of pyrimidine bases</u> (react with PPRP to form nucleotides):

| uracil | → | UMP |

| cytosine | → | CMP |

<u>Degradation of pyrimidine bases</u> (in liver):

Pyrimidine ring can be opened and completely degraded:

| cytosine | → CO_2, NH_4^+ and β-alanine

| thymine | → CO_2, NH_4^+ and β-aminoisobutyrate

These degradation products are harmless and excreted in the urine.

4.43.) <u>GENE EXPRESSION</u>

<u>BACTERIA (PROKARYOTES)</u>:

operon (DNA)	- operational unit that is either "on" or "off" - consists of promoter, operator and one or more structural genes
promoter (DNA)	- RNA polymerase binds to promoter - located 5'-end of operon ("upstream")
operator (DNA)	- located between promoter and structural genes - binding site of repressors - if repressor binds to operator, the operon is "off" (polymerase can't proceed)
repressor (protein)	- regulatory protein that binds to operator and prevents transcription
regulator gene (DNA)	- codes for repressor

---

lac-OPERON:
- *Metabolite (lactose) binds to repressor preventing its interaction with DNA.*
- *Operon freed of repressor is switched "on" and polymerase begins transcription of structural genes.*
- *Gene products: β-galactosidase and two other proteins*

HUMANS (EUKARYOTES):

- No operon. Each structural gene has its own promoter containing many different response elements (binding sites for regulatory proteins).

- Regulatory proteins can bind to several promoters activating a set of structural genes (which may be located on different chromosomes).

- Transcription is regulated by various combinations of regulatory proteins.

transcription factor	- binds to TATA box (part of promoter) - RNA polymerase does not recognize promoter in absence of transcription factor!
inducers	- *example: steroid hormones* - bind to nuclear receptor protein - inducer-receptor complex binds to DNA and activates some gene, inactivates others
enhancers	- regulatory DNA sequence - can be upstream or downstream of promoter - may be located several thousand base pairs from starting point of transcription - loops in DNA bring enhancers near the promoter region of the gene

4.44.) <u>TRANSCRIPTION</u>
DNA → RNA

<u>BACTERIA (PROKARYOTES):</u>

holoenzyme	- core enzyme plus σ-factor
σ-factors	- bind to RNA polymerase. - depending on σ-factor, RNA polymerase recognizes certain promoters but not others
cistron	- region of DNA that encodes a single protein

 Prokaryotic mRNA is polycistronic (encodes multiple proteins).

<u>HUMANS (EUKARYOTES):</u>

polymerase I	- makes rRNA
polymerase II	- makes mRNA
polymerase III	- makes tRNA

 Eukaryotic mRNA is heavily processed in the nucleus:
1. *5'-cap (methylated GTP) is added.*
2. *Poly (A) tail is added to 3' end.*
3. *Introns are removed and exons are spliced together.*

4.45.) <u>REPLICATION</u>
DNA → DNA

> - Parental strand is read in 3' to 5' direction.
> - New strand is produced in 5' to 3' direction.

 DNA polymerases cannot initiate synthesis of a new strand but require a primer (short oligonucleotide sequence composed of RNA). The primer is later replaced by DNA.

BACTERIA (PROKARYOTES):

helicase	- separates parental DNA
primase	- RNA polymerase that copies parental strand and makes RNA primer
polymerase III	- major DNA polymerase - replicates both parental strands - has proofreading ability - has 3' exonuclease activity to remove wrong nucleotides
polymerase I	- removes primer and fills gap with DNA (5' exonuclease activity)
polymerase II	- DNA repair (3' exonuclease activity)
ligase	- joins Okazaki fragments of lagging strand

HUMANS (EUKARYOTES):

δ	- major DNA polymerase - produces leading strand - also has helicase activity! - *no proofreading* - *no exonuclease activity*
α	- DNA polymerase - produces lagging strand - also has primase activity!
β, ε	- minor DNA polymerases - DNA repair (3' exonuclease activity)
γ	- mitochondrial DNA polymerase
ligase	- joins Okazaki fragments of lagging strand

Endonuclease: *Incision of DNA*
Exonuclease: *Removal of nucleotides from incised end*

ANATOMY

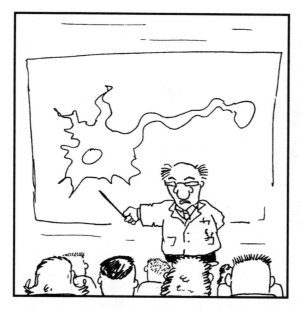

"There are 14 billion neurons in the brain and
14 billion *and one* facts to remember to pass
the Boards."

Part A : Embryology

5.1.) <u>GERM LAYERS</u>

ECTODERM	**neural tube** → CNS **neural crest** → peripheral nervous system **placodes** → sensory organs **surface epithelium** → skin
MESODERM	**somites** → muscles, vertebral column connective tissue lymphatic tissues
ENDODERM	epithelium of GI tract liver pancreas thymus thyroid

5.2.) <u>FETAL REMNANTS</u>

epigastric arteries	lateral umbilical ligaments
umbilical arteries	medial umbilical ligaments
urachus	median umbilical ligament
umbilical vein	round ligament
ductus venosus	venous ligament
ductus arteriosus	ligamentum arteriosus
yolk stalk	Meckel's diverticulum

<u>Meckel's diverticulum:</u>
- persists in 2% of persons
- located at antimesenteric border of ileum (within 2 feet of the ileocecal junction)
- inflammation may mimic appendicitis!

5.3.) DERIVATES OF BRANCHIAL ARCHES

	bones	muscles	arteries	nerves
1st Arch mandibular arch (Meckel)	malleus incus	muscles of mastication	facial artery	V3
2nd Arch hyoid arch (Reichert)	stapes styloid lesser horns of hyoid	muscles of facial expression	ext. carotid artery	VII
3rd Arch thyrohyoid arch	body of hyoid	stylopharyngeal muscle	int. carotid artery	IX
4th Arch	larynx	pharyngeal muscles		X

PHARYNGEAL CLEFTS:

I : (between arch I and II) forms external auditory meatus

II-IV : cervical sinus (disappears, but may form cervical cysts)

5.4.) <u>PHARYNGEAL POUCHES</u>

Each pharyngeal cleft has a corresponding pouch on the inside.
The clefts disappear (except for I), the pouches give of specialized tissues:

	tissues
I	tympanic cavity eustachian tube
II	palatine tonsil
III	ventral : thymus dorsal : <u>inferior</u> parathyroids
IV	ventral : - dorsal : <u>superior</u> parathyroids
V	ultimobranchial body (parafollicular C cells of thyroid)

<u>Cervical cysts:</u>
- *uncommon remnants of pharyngeal clefts*
- *located in anterolateral part of neck*
- *1-2 inches in diameter*

5.5.) <u>UROGENITAL DEVELOPMENT</u>

	male	female
Wolff	- **epididymis** - **vas deferens**	disappears
Müller	disappears	- **fallopian tubes** - **uterus** - **vagina down to hymen**

> ***Wolff*** *is sustained by testosterone (from Leydig cells)*
> ***Müller*** *is suppressed by MIF glycoprotein (from Sertoli cells)*

allantois	- **urinary bladder** - **urachus**
ureteric bud	- **bladder trigonum** - **ureter** - **collecting tubules**
pronephros	- disappears, never functional
mesonephros	- disappears, was functional
metanephros	- **kidneys**

Wolff: also called mesonephric duct
Müller: also called paramesonephric duct

Ureteric bud*: inferior part of mesonephric duct (= metanephric duct)*

Part B : Gross Anatomy

5.6.) <u>THE SKULL AND ITS HOLES</u>

optic canal	optic nerve ophthalmic artery
superior orbital fissure	cranial nerves III, IV, V (ophthalmic), VI sympathetic nerves opthalmic veins
foramen rotundum	cranial nerve V (maxillary)
foramen ovale	cranial nerve V (mandibular) accessory meningeal artery
foramen spinosum	middle meningeal artery
foramen magnum	spinal cord accessory nerve vertebral arteries spinal arteries
jugular foramen	cranial nerves IX, X, XI internal jugular vein
hypoglossal canal	cranial nerve XII
internal auditory meatus	cranial nerves VII, VIII labyrinthine artery

 Basilar skull fractures: Periorbital bruises or over mastoid process.

5.7.) <u>EYE</u>

A) <u>EXTERNAL MUSCLES</u>:

MUSCLE	MOVES EYE:	INNERVATION
med. rectus	nasal	III
lat. rectus	temporal	VI (abducens)
sup. rectus	up and nasal rotates medially	III
sup. oblique	down and temporal rotates medially	IV (trochlear)
inf. rectus	down and nasal rotates laterally	III
inf. oblique	up and temporal rotates laterally	III

 Abducens paralysis*: -> unable to abduct eye on affected side*
-> diplopia (double vision)

- <u>to raise eyes directly upwards:</u>
  needs combined action of superior rectus + inferior oblique

- <u>to depress eyes directly down:</u>
  needs combine action of inferior rectus + superior oblique

B) <u>INTERNAL MUSCLES</u>:

	FUNCTION	**INNERVATION**
dilator pupillae	mydriasis	sympathetic
sphincter pupillae	miosis	parasympathetic
ciliary	accommodation	parasympathetic

Contraction of the ciliary muscle relaxes suspensory ligaments and allows lens to turn into globular shape.

C) <u>UPPER EYELIDS</u>:

	FUNCTION	**INNERVATION**
levator palpebrae sup.	raises lid	III
Müller's muscle	raises lid	sympathetic

Drowsiness -> reduced sympathetic tone
  -> Müller's muscle relaxes
  -> eyelids droop

<u>HORNER'S SYNDROME</u>:
- neck injuries or tumors interrupting cervical sympathetic chain
- *miosis* (small pupils)
- *ptosis* (drooping eyelid)
- red and dry facial skin on affected side

5.8.) <u>TONGUE</u>

A) <u>MUSCLES</u>:

All tongue muscles are innervated by hypoglossal nerve (XII).

MUSCLES	FUNCTION
genioglossus	pulls it out
styloglossus	retracts it
hyoglossus	pulls it down

<u>DAMAGE TO HYPOGLOSSAL NERVE (XII)</u>:
- genioglossus muscle of healthy side becomes dominant
- tongue will deviate <u>towards</u> side of damage

B) <u>SENSATION</u>:

	TASTE	TOUCH, TEMPERATURE
anterior 2/3	VII	V3
posterior 1/3	IX	IX

5.9.) <u>MANDIBLE</u>

MUSCLES	FUNCTION
lat. pterygoid **digastric** **geniohyoid**	open mouth
masseter **medial pterygoid** **temporalis**	close mouth
lateral pterygoid	protrudes mandible
temporalis	retracts mandible
lateral pterygoid	lateral displacement

 These muscles are derived from the 1ˢᵗ branchial arch.
-> innervated by cranial nerve V (mandibular).

 A blow to the jaw often fractures the neck of the mandible
and/or the region of the opposite canine tooth.

5.10.) <u>LARYNX</u>

A) <u>MUSCLES</u>:

	FUNCTION	INNERVATION
post. cricoarytenoid	opens glottis	recurrent nerve
lat. cricoarytenoid	closes glottis	recurrent nerve
cricothyroid	tightens vocal chords	sup. laryngeal nerve
thyroarytenoid	relaxes vocal chords	recurrent nerve

- **Left recurrent** nerve wraps around aortic arch
- **Right recurrent** nerve wraps around right subclavian artery

Recurrent nerves are vulnerable to injury:
- *thyroidectomy*
- *carotid endarterectomy*
- *other operations in anterior triangle of the neck*

B) <u>SENSATION</u>:

above glottis	sup. laryngeal nerve
below glottis	recurrent nerve

5.11.) <u>SHOULDER</u>

FUNCTION	MAIN MUSCLE	INNERVATION
adduction	pectoralis major	C5-T1
abduction	first 60 degrees: deltoid then: serratus anterior	long thoracic nerve
anteversion	deltoid	axillary nerve
retroversion	teres major	subscapular nerve
outward rotation	infraspinatus	suprascapular nerve
inward rotation	subscapular	subscapular nerve

"<u>Scapular winging</u>" (paralysis of anterior serratus muscle):
- due to damage to the *long thoracic nerve* (stab wounds, thoracic surgery)
- medial border of scapula stands out when the person presses his arm anteriorly against a wall

> **<u>ROTATOR CUFF</u> : supraspinatus   infraspinatus**
> **teres minor   subscapularis**
>
> - *Holds the head of humerus in glenoid cavity of scapula.*
> - *Injury results in instability of shoulder joint.*

 Inflammation of subacromial bursa -> pain intensifies by abduction.

5.12.) <u>BRACHIAL PLEXUS</u>

spinal rami	trunks	terminal nerves
C5 - C6	upper trunk	musculocutaneous nerve
C7	middle trunk	axillary nerve radial nerve median nerve
C8 - T1	lower trunk	ulnar nerve

⌐ ̣ ̣ ̣ ̣ ̣ ̣ ̣¬ = posterior cord

<u>COMMON INJURIES TO PLEXUS</u>:

upper brachial plexus injury	- forceful separation of neck and shoulder - motorcycle accidents, football tackling - arm hangs in medial rotation ("waiter's tip position")
posterior cord injury	- compression by too long crutches - radial nerve injury (wrist drop)
lower brachial plexus injury	- forceful pull of arm/shoulders (birth) - ulnar nerve injury

240

5.13.) BRACHIAL NERVE INJURIES

	nerve injury results in:
radial nerve	- wrist drop - loss of triceps reflex - *sensory loss: posterior arm, dorsal hand*
median nerve	- no flexion of thumb, index and middle finger - no thumb opposition - thenar atrophy - *sensory loss: palmar aspect first 3 fingers*
ulnar nerve	- claw hand - no flexion of 4th and 5th finger - apothenar atrophy - *sensory loss: 5th and lateral 4th finger*
musculocutaneous n.	- no elbow flexion - no supination - loss of biceps reflex

Carpal tunnel syndrome: *Compression of median nerve by carpal ligament.*
-> pain/tingling in distribution area of median nerve
(often most bothersome at night)

Humerus fracture: *Risk of radial nerve injury (spirals down near humerus).*

5.14.) <u>ELBOW</u>

FUNCTION	MAIN MUSCLE	INNERVATION
flexion	biceps brachii	musculocutaneous nerve
extension	triceps brachii	radial nerve
supination	biceps brachii	musculocutaneous nerve
pronation	pronator teres	median nerve

<u>"Tennis elbow"</u>:
- repetitive stress, especially "backhand play"
- due to inflammation of the lateral epicondyle, which is the origin of extensor muscles of the forearm.
- The elbow joint and olecranon are NOT involved!

Supination: palm faces anteriorly, thumb points to lateral side.
Pronation: palm faces posteriorly, thumb points to medial side.

Colles' fracture: Fracture of radius near wrist
-> dorsal/lateral position of hand

5.15.) <u>HIP</u>

FUNCTION	MAIN MUSCLES	INNERVATION
outward rotation	gluteus maximus	inf. gluteal nerve
inward rotation	gluteus medius / minimus	sup. gluteal nerve
extension	gluteus maximus	inf. gluteal nerve
flexion	iliopsoas	femoral nerve
abduction	gluteus medius	sup. gluteal nerve
adduction	adductor magnus / minimus	obturator nerve

 Femur neck fracture*: the leg is abducted and externally rotated.*

Pelvic fractures: - automobile accidents
- risk of severe internal bleeding

Femur neck fractures: - common in elderly women
(osteoporosis)
- risk of femur head necrosis
- significant morbidity / mortality

5.16.) <u>KNEE</u>

FUNCTION	MAIN MUSCLE	INNERVATION
extension	quadriceps femoris	femoral nerve
flexion	"<u>hamstrings</u>": - semimembranous muscle - semitendinous muscle - biceps femoris	sciatic nerve
inward rotation	semimembranous	sciatic nerve
outward rotation	biceps femoris	sciatic nerve

<u>**Pulled hamstrings:**</u>
- Common sports injury in persons who run and kick balls
- Tearing of fibers -> very painful

<u>**Knee injury:**</u>
- Rupture of anterior cruciate ligament: tibia can be drawn anteriorly.
- Rupture of posterior cruciate ligament: tibia can be drawn posteriorly.
- Rupture of lateral ligaments: tibia can be bend laterally.
- Meniscus injuries: pain upon extension of flexed knee (McMurray's test).

The gluteal region is a common side for IM injection of drugs.
- risk of sciatic nerve injury
- upper lateral quadrant is relatively safe

5.17.) ANKLE

Each muscle moves ankle in two axes:

MUSCLE	FUNCTION	INNERVATION
tibialis anterior	dorsiflexes + *inverts foot*	deep peroneal nerve
peroneus tertius	dorsiflexes + *everts foot*	deep peroneal nerve
peroneus longus and brevis	plantarflexes + *inverts foot*	superficial peroneal n.
tibialis posterior	plantarflexes + *everts foot*	tibial nerve

Injury to common peroneal nerve:
- winds around neck of fibula
- most commonly injured nerve of lower limb
- loss of dorsiflexion -> "foot drop"

Injury to tibial nerve:
- rare (deep laceration of popliteal fossa)
- inability to plantarflex foot and toes

Fractures of tibia:
- "bumper fractures"
- skin tears -> frequent compound fractures

5.18.) <u>MEDIASTINUM</u>

superior mediastinum	- thymus - great vessels of heart - trachea - esophagus
middle mediastinum	- heart
posterior (of heart) mediastinum	- esophagus - descending aorta
anterior (of heart) mediastinum	- large during infancy (filled by thymus)[1]

[1] in infancy is wider than the heart silhouette on X-ray!

5.19.) <u>CORONARY ARTERIES</u>

	supplies:
left coronary artery -> ant. interventricular and circumflex artery	left atrium left ventricle septum
right coronary artery	right atrium right ventricle variable amount of left atrium and ventricle sinus node AV node

 Blood flow *through coronary arteries is highest during early diastole and lowest during systole!*

5.20.) __ABDOMINAL ARTERIES__

	branches	organs
celiac trunk	left gastric artery splenic artery hepatic artery gastroduodenal artery sup. pancreaticoduodenal art.	stomach spleen liver proximal duodenum
sup. mesenteric art.	inf. pancreaticoduodenal art. many branches	distal duodenum small intestine cecum ascending colon transverse colon
inf. mesenteric art.	many branches superior rectal artery	descending colon sigmoid rectum

---

Portocaval shunts:
- gastric/esophageal veins -> esophageal varices
- anorectal veins   -> hemorrhoids
- paraumbilical veins   -> caput medusae

5.21.) <u>PERITONEUM</u>

intraperitoneal	retroperitoneal
stomach	aorta
small bowel	vena cava
transverse colon	kidneys
spleen	pancreas
(liver)	duodenum
	ascending colon
	descending colon

<u>**ACUTE APPENDICITIS:**</u>
McBurney's point: at junction between lateral and middle thirds of a line between umbilicus and anterior superior iliac spine

 <u>Signs of peritonitis:</u>
severe pain (localized or diffuse)
rebound tenderness
abdominal muscle rigidity

5.22.) <u>LAYERS OF SPERMATIC CORD</u>

deep

loose connective tissue	arteries, pampiniform plexus
internal spermatic fascia	from fascia transversalis
cremaster muscle and fascia	from int. oblique muscle
external spermatic fascia	from ext. oblique aponeurosis
superficial fascia	contains dartos muscle

superficial

5.23.) <u>OVARY / TESTIS</u>

"Important organs receive multiple blood supplies."

ovary	aorta -> ovarian artery internal iliac a. -> uterine artery
testis	aorta -> testicular artery internal iliac a. -> art. of ductus deferens inf. epigastric a. -> cremasteric artery

Part C : Neuroanatomy

5.24.) CORTEX

left hemisphere	right hemisphere
language	non-verbal
mathematics	musical
sequential	geometrical
analytical	spatial comprehension

vision	occipital lobe
hearing	temporal lobe
taste	insula, below postcentral gyrus
reading, writing	angular gyrus
primary motor cortex	precentral gyrus
primary sensory cortex	postcentral gyrus
Wernicke (sensory)	temporal lobe, superior gyrus
Broca (motor)	frontal lobe, near lateral fissure

APHASIAS:
- **Broca:** nonfluent speech, good comprehension
- **Wernicke:** fluent but nonsensical speech, poor comprehension

5.25.) CEREBRAL ARTERIES

Stroke: *80% ischemic, 20% hemorrhagic*

	supplies:	**occlusion results in:**
ophthalmic a.	eye	unilateral blindness
post. cerebral a.	occipital lobe	homonymous hemianopsia (contralateral)
middle cerebral a.	lateral cortex ant. limb of internal capsule	motor & sensory loss (upper body)
ant. cerebral a.	medial cortex	motor & sensory loss (legs and feet)
ant. choroidal a.	basal ganglia hypothalamus post. limb of internal capsule	
cerebellar aa.	cerebellum lateral portions of brain stem	ataxia brainstem syndromes

homonymous hemianopsia:

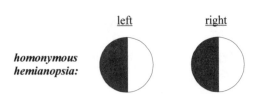

left   right

5.26.) <u>TRANSIENT ISCHEMIC ATTACKS</u>

internal carotid artery	vertebrobasilar artery
- ipsilateral monocular blindness ("amaurosis fugax") - hemiparesis, contralateral - hemisensory loss, contralateral - language disturbance	- vertigo - diplopia - ataxia - facial numbness/weakness - nausea

5.27.) <u>HYPERTENSIVE HEMORRHAGE</u>

hemorrhage into:	results in:
putamen	contralateral weakness, including face contralateral hemianopsia
thalamus	contralateral hemiparesis sensory changes homonymous hemianopsia
pons	coma small reactive pupils quadriplegia
cerebellum	unsteady gait clumsiness nausea, vomiting

5.28.) <u>CRANIAL NERVES</u>

	nerve	functions
somatic motor	III	extraocular eye muscles (except sup. oblique and lat. rectus)
	IV	superior oblique
	VI	lateral rectus
	XII	tongue muscles (except palatoglossus)
branchial motor (derived from branchial arches)	V	mastication
	VII	facial expression
	IX, X	pharynx, larynx
	XI	trapezius, sternocleidomastoid muscles
visceral motor	III	ciliary muscle, constrictor pupillae
	VII	all glands except parotid
	IX	parotid
	X	abdominal viscera up to splenic flexure
special sensory	I	smell
	II	vision
	VII, IX	taste
	VIII	hearing, balance
general sensory	V, VII, IX, X	pain, temperature, touch, proprioception
visceral sensory	IX, X	afferents for visceral reflexes

5.29.) <u>PARASYMPATHETIC GANGLIA</u>

Nucleus	Nerve	Ganglion	Organs
Edinger-Westphal	III	ciliary	eye
sup. salivary nucleus	VII	sublingual submaxillary	lacrimal gland nasal glands submandibular gland
inf. salivary nucleus	IX	otic	parotid gland
dorsal motor nucleus	X	many, mostly intramural	many

Pupillary light reflex: *Optical nerve → tectal area → Edinger-Westphal nucleus → parasympathetic → sphincter*
Argyll-Robertson pupil: *Damage to tectal area (e.g. syphilis): pupils constrict for near vision but not for light.*

255

5.30.) <u>BASAL GANGLIA</u>

striatum	caudate putamen globus pallidum
neostriatum	caudate putamen
paleostriatum	globus pallidum
lentiform nucleus	putamen globus pallidum

<u>Parkinson's disease:</u>
- loss of dopaminergic input from substantia nigra to striatum
- -> bradykinesia (difficulty initiating or stopping a movement)
- -> muscle rigidity
- -> tremor ("pill-rolling")

<u>Huntington's disease:</u>
- atrophy of caudate nucleus
- -> chorea: involuntary movements
- personality changes, dementia

<u>Wilson's disease:</u>
- copper accumulation in lentiform nucleus (and elsewhere)
- -> tremor, spasticity, chorea, bizarre behavior

5.31.) THALAMUS

> **"Thalamus knows all" (receives all sensory input, except olfactory)**

I.) ANTERIOR THALAMUS (part of limbic system)	input : mammillary bodies output : cingula (cortex)
II.) LATERAL THALAMUS	major nucleus: "pulvinar"
ventral anterior nucleus	receives input from basal ganglia output to premotor cortex

ventral posterior nucleus	**VPL** : medial lemniscus, spinothalamic tract
	      (proprioception, touch)
	VPM : trigeminal nerve
	      (taste)

ventrolateral nucleus	input from cerebellum and basal ganglia output to motor cortex
III.) MEDIAL THALAMUS	projects to frontal cortex
IV.) POSTERIOR THALAMUS	**medial geniculate:** auditory pathway **lateral geniculate:** optic tract

---

General features of thalamus:
- major synaptic relay station (sensory input)
- basal ganglia -> thalamus -> cortex
- rhythm established by thalamus forms major contribution to EEG

Some patients with thalamic injury become insensitive to pain and other sensory stimuli.

5.32.) BRAINSTEM SYNDROMES

	blood supply
medulla	**lateral:** posterior inferior cerebellar artery **medial:** anterior spinal artery
lower pons	**lateral:** anterior inferior cerebellar artery **medial:** basilar artery
upper pons	**lateral:** superior cerebellar artery **medial:** basilar artery

- Brainstem syndromes are complex because many structures are packed tightly together in a small space.
- The most famous one is the Wallenberg syndrome (lateral medulla infarction due to occlusion of posterior inferior cerebellar artery).

5.33.) MEDULLA

Infarction of lateral medulla:

DAMAGE TO:	RESULTS IN:
spinal tract nucleus V	ipsilateral face: pain / temp loss
nucleus solitarius	ipsilateral tongue: loss of taste
reticular formation	ipsilateral Horner's syndrome
nucleus ambiguus	hoarseness loss of pharyngeal reflex
spinothalamic tract	contralateral body pain / temp loss

Infarction of medial medulla:

DAMAGE TO:	RESULTS IN:
hypoglossal muscle	ipsilateral tongue: atrophic paralysis
medial lemniscus	contralateral loss of position sense contralateral loss of vibration sense
pyramidal tract	contralateral body: spastic paralysis

5.34.) <u>LOWER PONS</u>

<u>Infarction of lateral pons:</u>

DAMAGE TO:	RESULTS IN:
spinocerebellar tract	ipsilateral limb ataxia
nucleus VII	ipsilateral face: paralysis
spinal tract nucleus V	ipsilateral face: loss of sensation
reticular formation	ipsilateral Horner's syndrome
vestibular nucleus	vertigo
cochlear nuclei	deafness / tinnitus

<u>Infarction of medial pons:</u>

DAMAGE TO:	RESULTS IN:
nucleus VII	ipsilateral face: spastic paralysis
medial long. fasciculus	ipsilateral eye can not adduct on lateral gaze
nucleus VI	ipsilateral paralysis of lat. rectus oculi
corticospinal tract	contralateral body: spastic paralysis
medial lemniscus	contralateral loss of position and vibration sense

5.35.) UPPER PONS

Infarction of lateral pons:

DAMAGE TO:	RESULTS IN:
motor nucleus V	ipsilateral loss of masseter function
reticular formation	ipsilateral Horner's syndrome
spinothalamic tract	contralateral loss of pain and sensation

Infarction of medial pons:

DAMAGE TO:	RESULTS IN:
corticospinal tract	contralateral spastic paralysis

5.36.) <u>WHERE IS THE LESION?</u>

SYMPTOMS	LESION
Loss of pain and temperature sensation arms and shoulder	Syringomyelia
Muscle weakness and loss of sensation in left arm	Right middle cerebral a.
Muscle weakness and loss of sensation in left leg	Right anterior cerebral a.
Spastic paralysis, loss of proprioception left leg and loss of pain and temperature sensation right leg	Hemisection of left spinal cord
Spastic paralysis both legs	Total transection of spinal cord
Flaccid paralysis, loss of sensations, both legs	Guillain-Barré syndrome
Muscle atrophy, fasciculations both arms & legs	ALS
Loss of pain and temperature sensation left arms, legs, body, paralysis of left arms, legs and body and loss of sensation right lower face	"Wallenberg syndrome" (right lateral medulla)
Sensory loss both hands and feet ("sock&glove pattern")	Peripheral neuropathy
Loss of sensation over buttocks, perineum and impotence	Cauda equina lesion

5.37.) <u>KEY DERMATOMES</u>

skull	C2
thumb	C6
nipple	T5
belly button	T10
big toe	L4
penis	S3
anus	S5
knee jerk reflex	**L4**
ankle jerk reflex	**S1**

PHYSIOLOGY

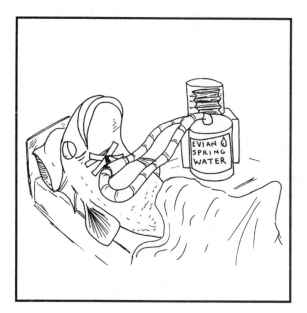

Fish respirators.

6.1.) <u>SIX EQUATIONS YOU REALLY NEED</u>

1. HOW TO CALCULATE TOTAL PERIPHERAL RESISTANCE:

Mean blood pressure $\qquad P_{average} = P_{diastolic} + 1/3\ (P_{systolic} - P_{diastolic})$

Total peripheral resistance $\qquad$ TPR = mean blood pressure / cardiac output

EXAMPLE: $\qquad$ systolic blood pressure 120 mmHg
$\qquad\qquad\qquad$ diastolic blood pressure 80 mmHg
$\qquad\qquad\qquad$ cardiac output 5,000 mL/min

$\qquad\qquad\qquad$ -> mean pressure = 80 +1/3 (120-80) = 93 mmHg
$\qquad\qquad\qquad$ -> TPR = 93/5,000 = 0.018

Norepinephrine increases TPR (α-receptors -> vasoconstriction)
Epinephrine decreases TPR (β-receptors -> vasodilation)

2. HOW TO CALCULATE CARDIAC OUTPUT:

Cardiac output = systemic blood flow = pulmonary blood flow
(Assuming that there are no intracardiac shunts!)

Fick's Principle: $\quad$ pulmonary flow = oxygen uptake / (a-v oxygen difference)

EXAMPLE: $\qquad$ arterial O_2 = 20 mL oxygen / 100 mL blood = 0.2
$\qquad\qquad\qquad$ venous O_2 = 15 mL oxygen / 100 mL blood = 0.15
$\qquad\qquad\qquad$ oxygen uptake = 250 mL / min

$\qquad\qquad\qquad$ -> cardiac output = 250 / 0.05 = 5,000 mL / min

Cardiac output is usually normalized by body surface area (= "cardiac index").

3. HOW TO CALCULATE RENAL CLEARANCE:

Clearance of X   clearance · $[X]_{plasma}$ = urine flow · $[X]_{urine}$

EXAMPLE: plasma creatinine concentration = 1.5 mg/dL
urine creatinine concentration = 180 mg/dL
urine flow = 1,500 mL / 24 h ≈ 1 mL/min

-> creatinine clearance = 1 mL/min (180/1.5) = 120 mL/min

4. ACID / BASE CALCULATIONS:

Henderson-Hasselbalch $pH = pK + \log \dfrac{[salt]}{[acid]}$

$$pH = 6.1 + \log \dfrac{[HCO_3^-]}{[CO_2]}$$

$$pH = 6.1 + \log \dfrac{[HCO_3^-]}{0.03 \; PCO_2}$$

EXAMPLE: plasma bicarbonate = 24 mM/L
PCO_2 = 40 mmHg

-> pH = 6.1 + log (24/1.2) = 6.1 + log (20) = 7.4

Bicarbonate is a powerful buffer (despite having a pK 6.1 far from physiological pH) because the acid (H_2CO_3 <-> CO_2) and salt (HCO_3^-) concentrations are independently regulated by the body:

- *Kidneys regulate HCO_3^-*
- *Lung ventilation regulates CO_2*

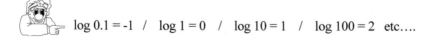 log 0.1 = -1 / log 1 = 0 / log 10 = 1 / log 100 = 2 etc....

5. HOW TO CALCULATE DIFFUSION CAPACITY OF THE LUNG:

Diffusion (Fick's law) $flow = D \cdot area \cdot \dfrac{concentration\ gradient}{membrane\ thickness}$

Since lung area and membrane thickness of the lung cannot be measured directly, they are lumped together with the diffusion coefficient:

$$flow = D_L \cdot concentration\ gradient$$

EXAMPLE: alveolar partial pressure of CO = 200 mmHg
blood partial pressure of CO = 0 mmHg
flow = 4,000 mL/min

-> CO diffusion capacity $D_{L_{CO}}$ = 20 mL / min $\cdot$ mmHg

CO_2 and O_2 equilibrate within $1/3^{rd}$ of capillary transient time (<u>perfusion limited!</u>)

CO on the other hand is less lipid soluble (<u>diffusion limited</u>) and therefore well suited for measuring diffusion properties of the lung. This is done with a single inspiration of diluted CO and measuring the rate of disappearance of CO from alveolar gas.

Increased D_L: Recruitment and dilation of pulmonary capillaries.
(may double during exercise!)

Decreased D_L: Interstitial lung diseases, emphysema and V/Q imbalance.

6. HOW TO CALCULATE LUNG COMPLIANCE:

Elasticity $elasticity = \dfrac{\Delta\ pressure}{\Delta\ volume}$

Compliance ("stretchability") $compliance = 1/elasticity = \dfrac{\Delta\ volume}{\Delta\ pressure}$

Patient's with COPD have lungs with <u>high</u> compliance.
Patient's with restrictive lung disease have <u>low</u> compliance.
A rod of steal has higher elasticity (less stretchability) than a rubber band.

6.2.) <u>ION CHANNELS</u>

	key features
K^+ channels	- maintain resting membrane potential - repolarization phase of action potentials - afterhyperpolarization
Na^+ channels	- upstroke phase of action potential - rapid inactivation -> repolarization (refractory period)
Ca^{2+} channels	- excitation contraction coupling - excitation secretion coupling - cardiac pacemaker potential (sinus node) - cardiac plateau phase: Ca^{2+} entry - intracellular Ca^{2+} release (ryanodine receptor)
cation channels	- depolarization - dark current of photoreceptors - ACh receptor at motor endplate
Cl^- channels	- CNS: inhibitory postsynaptic potentials
Na^+ / K^+ pump	- maintains ion gradients - is electrogenic (but direct contribution to RMP is very small)

Absolute refractory phase:
Action potentials cannot be generated because of inactivation of the Na^+ channels.

Relative refractory phase:
Some Na^+ channels have recovered from inactivation. Strong stimuli may generate action potentials with slow upstroke and low amplitude.

6.3.) <u>TRANSPORT</u>

	passive	facilitated	active
ATP required?	no	no	yes
can it transport against gradient?	no	no (yes if coupled)	yes
substrate specific?	no	yes	yes
saturating?	no	yes	yes

<u>EXAMPLES:</u>

- Active transport: Na^+ / K^+ ATPase
  H^+ / K^+ ATPase

- Facilitated transport: simple glucose carriers

  Secondary active transport: $Na^+ /$ glucose carriers
  $Na^+ /$ amino acid carriers

  (In this case, glucose and amino acids are transported <u>against</u> their gradients, but this is driven by Na^+ moving down its own gradient.)

- Passive transport: water, electrolytes, O_2 etc.

6.4.) <u>SIGNAL TRANSDUCTION</u>

	hormones / receptors
IP3, DAG	α1, M1, M4, H1 angiotensin II tachykinins endothelin
cAMP ↑	β, H2 ACTH
cAMP ↓	α2 M2, M3
cGMP ↑	EDRF (nitric oxide) ANP Viagra®[1]
tyrosine kinase	insulin growth factors
gene expression	steroid hormones thyroid hormones retinoic acid

[1] inhibits type V cGMP phosphodiesterase -> enhanced effect of nitric oxide on penile artery dilation.

***Tyrosine kinase** phosphorylates many proteins. It also activates the ras -> raf -> MAP kinase cascade which modulates gene expression. Out of control activation of ras is a/w with many neoplasms.*

G proteins function like a timer mechanism:
- Hormone receptor interaction first sets the timer (GDP on α-subunit is replaced by GTP), then starts it (α-subunit dissociates from β/γ).
- Activated α-subunit interacts with other enzymes such as adenylate cyclase.
- α-subunit has built-in enzymatic activity that hydrolyzes its GTP to GDP, which terminates the action of the α-subunit ("time is out").

Gi	inhibits adenylate cyclase
Go	stimulates adenylate cyclase
Gq	activates phospholipase C

6.5.) NERVE FIBERS

large diameter high velocity		
	Aα	- efferent: skeletal muscle - afferent: from muscle spindle
	Aγ	- efferent: to muscle spindle
	Aβ , Aδ	- afferent: touch fast sharp pain
	C	- afferent: slow dull pain
small diameter low velocity	**B , C**	- efferent: autonomic nerves

"All-or-None" response:
If the stimulus is not strong enough to depolarize the membrane to threshold, no action potential occurs. If threshold is reached, a uniform action potential is generated. Stimulus strength determines frequency of action potential generation.

6.6.) <u>TOUCH RECEPTORS</u>

pressure	Merkel's disks *(slowly adapting)*	
touch	Meissner's corpuscle *(fast adapting)* hair follicle sensors	
vibration	Pacinian corpuscle *(most rapidly adapting)*	
pain and temperature	mostly free nerve endings	

Paradoxical cold: *At temperatures > 45°C (120F) cold fibers begin to fire again (together with pain fibers). This sensation of pain and coolness is called "paradoxical cold".*

6.7.) <u>ACCOMMODATION</u>

near object	far object
ciliary muscle contracted	ciliary muscle relaxed
zonula fibers relaxed	zonula fibers tense
lens rounded (if elastic)	lens flat
focal length short	focal length far

myopia (nearsightedness)	- lens has normal elasticity - focal point too short (or eye ball too long) - *corrected with negative lens (concave)*
hypermetropia (farsightedness)	- lens has normal elasticity - focal point too far (or eye ball too short) - *corrected with positive lens (convex)*
presbyopia (age)	- lens has lost elasticity - cannot shorten focal length - *corrected with positive lens (convex)*

Patients with hypermetropia and presbyopia have difficulty reading.

6.8.) <u>NYSTAGMUS</u>

| Direction of nystagmus is defined by the <u>fast</u> phase. |

optokinetic	- looking out of train *nystagmus against movement of image*
vestibular	- postrotational nystagmus *nystagmus against direction of prior rotation* - caloric nystagmus *nystagmus away from cold ear*

 Caloric testing is used to diagnose labyrinthine disease (vertigo).

6.9.) <u>COCHLEA</u>

scala vestibuli	Na$^+$ rich	perilymph
scala media	K$^+$ rich	endolymph
scala tympani	Na$^+$ rich	perilymph

- *Basilar membrane is between media and tympani.*
- *Endocochlear potential: Scala media = +80 mV*

6.10.) DEAFNESS

TUNING FORK TESTS:

	Weber	Rinne
method	Place fork on top of skull	Place fork on mastoid process until tone disappears (= bone conduction). Then hold next to ear (= air conduction).
normal	Sound is equal in both ears.	Air conduction is better than bone conduction.
conduction deafness [1] (middle ear)	Sound lateralized to sick ear.	Bone conduction is better than air conduction.
nerve deafness [2] (inner ear)	Sound lateralized to normal ear.	Air conduction is better than bone conduction.

[1] chronic otitis, otosclerosis or occlusion of external auditory meatus
[2] cochlear disease or injury to cranial nerve VIII.

 Unilateral cortical lesions do NOT affect hearing since cochlear nuclei project to both temporal lobes.

6.11.) <u>AUTONOMIC NERVOUS SYSTEM</u>

	sympathetic	parasympathetic
heart	increased heart rate increased conduction increased force	decreased heart rate
bronchi	dilates	constricts
GI tract	reduces motility	increases motility
sphincters of GI tract	constricts	relaxes
rectum	allows filling	empties relaxes internal sphincter
bladder	allows filling	empties relaxes internal sphincter
erection		maintains erection
ejaculation	triggers ejaculation	
pupils of eye	big (mydriasis)	small (miosis)
sweat glands	sweat (cholinergic!)	
salivary glands		secretion
blood vessels	depends on receptors: - α constricts - β dilates	no direct effect (except artery of penis)

<u>Four ways to decrease blood pressure:</u>
- block nicotinic ganglionic receptors
- block β receptors
- block α1 receptors
- stimulate α2 receptors

6.12.) <u>MUSCARINIC RECEPTORS</u>

	location

nicotinic	- **autonomic ganglia**
	  sympathetic and parasympathetic ganglia!
	- adrenal medulla
	
	- **neuromuscular junction**
	  these receptors differ from autonomic ones!

muscarinic	- **postsynaptic parasympathetic** - **sweat glands** (innervated by sympathetic nerves!) - *second messenger depends on receptor subtype:* *M1, M3 -> PLC -> IP3, DAG* *M2, M4 -> inhibit adenylate cyclase -> cAMP↓* * open K^+ channels*

Antagonists: *Nicotinic (ganglionic):* hexamethonium
Nicotinic (motor endplate): tubocurarine
Muscarinic: atropine

6.13.) ADRENERGIC RECEPTORS

alpha 1	**- postsynaptic sympathetic**
	    generally excitatory (vasoconstriction)
	    in GI tract inhibitory
	
	- Gq -> phospholipase C -> IP3, DAG

alpha 2	**- presynaptic sympathetic**
	    (decrease catecholamine release)
	
	- central nervous system
	    (decrease sympathetic tone)
	
	- Gi -> inhibits adenylate cyclase -> cAMP↓

beta 1	**- postsynaptic sympathetic (cardiac)** excitatory (chronotrope, dromotrope, inotrope) *Gs -> adenylate cyclase -> cAMP↑*
beta 2	**- postsynaptic sympathetic (all others)** inhibitory (vasodilation, bronchodilation) *Gs -> adenylate cyclase -> cAMP↑*

Agonists: *alpha: epinephrine ≥ norepinephrine >> isoproterenol*
                beta 1 : isoproterenol > epinephrine = norepinephrine
                beta 2 : isoproterenol > epinephrine >> norepinephrine

---

Vascular tone:
- Norepinephrine injection -> stimulates α-receptors -> vasoconstriction -> increase in diastolic blood pressure.
- Epinephrine injection -> stimulates α and β-receptors, but β-effect predominates -> vasodilation -> decrease in diastolic blood pressure.

6.14.) <u>CONTROL OF HEART BEAT</u>

right vagus nerve	- slows frequency (sinus node)
left vagus nerve	- slows conduction (AV node) - decreased force of contraction (atria but not ventricles!)
sympathetic	- increased frequency - increased conduction - increased force of contraction (atria and ventricles)
epinephrine injection	- increased conduction and contraction - increased frequency - *increased systolic pressure* - *decreased diastolic pressure (vasodilation)*
norepinephrine injection	- increased conduction and contraction - decreased frequency (baroreceptor reflex !) - *increased systolic pressure* - *increased diastolic pressure (vasoconstriction)*

<u>**Frank Starling mechanism:**</u>
Preload = end-diastolic volume in ventricle
Preload↑ -> muscle filament overlap↑ -> stroke volume↑

6.15.) <u>CONTROL OF MUSCLE TONE</u>

	function	nerve fiber
muscle spindle	- measures muscle <u>length</u> - activates α motoneuron when stretched	γ efferent 1A afferent
Golgi tendon organ	- measures muscle <u>tension</u> - inhibits α motoneuron	1B afferent

Stretch reflex (for example knee jerk reflex): Intrafusal fibers (muscle spindle) are parallel with skeletal muscle fibers. Stretching results in firing of 1A afferent that excites the α-motoneuron (monosynaptic reflex). The α-motoneuron of the antagonistic muscle is inhibited via an interneuron.

Increased muscle tone:
- activation of γ fibers
- upper motor neuron lesions (hemiplegia)
- Parkinson
- cold, anxiety

Decreased muscle tone:
- lower motor neuron lesions
- spinal shock (early phase of hemiplegia)
- warmth

Decorticate posture:
- legs extended, arms flexed (cortex injury)

Decerebrate posture:
- legs and arms extended (brainstem injury)

6.16.) <u>MUSCLE TYPES</u>

	RED SKELETAL MUSCLE	WHITE SKELETAL MUSCLE
myosin isoenzyme	**slow**	**fast**
glycolytic capacity	low	high
oxidative capacity	high	low

oxidative capacity <u>related to</u>
- number of capillaries
- myoglobin content
- number of mitochondria

6.17.) <u>ELECTROMECHANICAL COUPLING</u>

skeletal muscle	heart muscle	smooth muscle
motor units [1]	syncytium	syncytium
action potential: 2-4 ms	action potential: 200-400 ms	<u>tonic</u> - vascular smooth muscle <u>phasic</u> - visceral smooth muscle - slow waves, spikes
Ca^{2+} binds to troponin	Ca^{2+} binds to troponin	Ca^{2+} -calmodulin -> MLC phosphorylation
Ca^{2+} release from SR	Ca^{2+} influx	Ca^{2+} influx and release
tetanus	no tetanus	myogenic tone

[1] motor unit = all muscle fibers innervated by same α-motoneuron

<u>REGULATION OF FORCE:</u>

skeletal muscle	heart muscle	smooth muscle
- recruitment of motor units - AP frequency	- AP duration	- membrane potential - biochemical modulation of Ca^{2+} sensitivity

6.18.) <u>CARDIAC CYCLE</u>

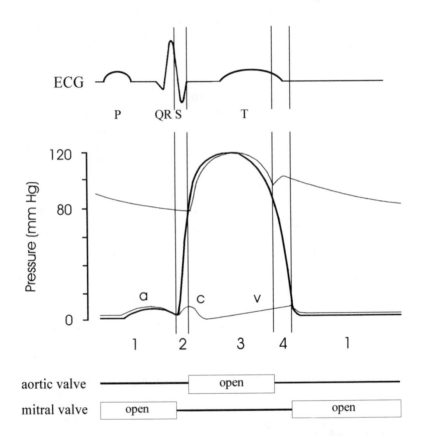

1 - filling
2 - isovolumetric contraction
3 - ejection
4 - isovolumetric relaxation

a-wave : atrial contraction
c-wave : bulging of mitral valve
v-wave : filling of atria

6.19.) <u>LUNG VOLUMES</u>

IRV	= 3.0L
IV	= 0.5L
ERV	= 1.2L
RV	= 1.3L

IC	= 3.5L
FRC	= 2.5L

VC = 4.7L

TC = 6.0L

IRV, IV and ERV are measured by spirometer
RV is measured by helium dilution or body plethysmography

- Ventilation = dV/dt
- Alveolar ventilation = ventilation - dead space ventilation

Dead is space measured by nitrogen exhalation
(inhale 100% oxygen, measure N_2 while exhaling)

- Dead space = anatomical dead space plus unperfused alveoli
- Ventilated alveoli that are unperfused (for example pulmonary embolus) increase dead space. This situation s called V/Q mismatch.

<u>Ventilation / Perfusion ratio V/Q</u>
V is higher at **base** of lung than at tip.
Q is higher at **base** of lung than at tip.
V/Q is higher at **tip** of lung than at base!

(That's why tubercle bacilli are found at tips of lung,
while pneumonia tends to develop at base of lungs.)

	obstructive	restrictive
VC	↓	↓
FRC, RV	↑	↓
TC	∅ or ↑	↓

6.20.) __BREATHING PATTERNS__

Cheyne-Stokes	- **waxing and waning** - uremia - can be physiological at high altitude
Kussmaul	- **deep, fast inspirations** - compensation of metabolic acidosis (e.g. diabetic ketoacidosis)
Biot	- **apneic episodes** - brain tumors

__Chronic lung disease (COPD):__
-> central CO_2 receptors become less responsive.
-> peripheral O_2 receptors become "more important".
-> do not administer pure O_2 (or patient may stop breathing!)

EXPERIMENTAL TRANSSECTIONS:

above pons	normal respiration continues
above pons plus vagotomy	deeper inspirations (removal of afferent input from pulmonary sensory receptors)
mid pons	same effect as vagotomy
mid pons plus vagotomy	"apneusis" = arrested in inspiratory state [1]
below pons	irregular, fast and deep respiration (like gasping)
below medulla	all respirations seize

[1] *this finding is taken as evidence for a "pneumotaxic center" located in the rostral pons which functions to limit the extent of inspirations.*

6.21.) <u>RESPIRATORY QUOTIENT</u>
(CO_2 release / O_2 uptake)

	kcal / g	RQ
carbohydrates	4	1.0
proteins	4	0.8
fat	9	0.7

RQ < 0.7	- hypoventilation - diabetes - fasting
RQ > 1.0	- hyperventilation

6.22.) ACID BASE

	pH	primary disturbance	compensatory response	clinical conditions
respiratory acidosis	< 7.35	PCO_2 ↑	HCO_3^- ↑	- sedation - sleep apnea - chest wall injuries - COPD
metabolic acidosis	< 7.35	HCO_3^- ↓	PCO_2 ↓	- ketoacidosis (diabetes) - lactacidosis (shock) - chronic diarrhea
respiratory alkalosis	> 7.45	PCO_2 ↓	HCO_3^- ↓	- anxiety - thyrotoxicosis - mountain climbing
metabolic alkalosis	> 7.45	HCO_3^- ↑	PCO_2 ↑	- loop diuretics (K^+ loss) - insulin (K^+ redistribution) - vomiting (H^+ loss)

SALICYLATE INTOXICATION:
Early: metabolic acidosis + respiratory alkalosis
Late: metabolic acidosis + respiratory acidosis

6.23.) <u>HEMOGLOBINS</u>

	hemoglobin	chains
embryo	Gower 1	$\zeta_2\varepsilon_2$
fetus	HbF	$\alpha_2\gamma_2$
adult	HbA HbA$_2$ HbA$_{1C}$	$\alpha_2\beta_2$ (98%) $\alpha_2\delta_2$ (2%) glycosylated derivative
sickle cell anemia	HbS	$\alpha_2\beta^S_2$
α-thalassemia	HbH Hb Bart	β_4 γ_4
β-thalassemia	HbF HbA$_2$	$\alpha_2\delta_2$ $\alpha_2\gamma_2$

Sickle cell anemia is due to a point mutation of the β-chains. HbS forms polymers on deoxygenation, red cells loose their deformability and assume a sickled shape.

Hemoglobin is a major H^+ buffer of the blood. Deoxygenated hemoglobin is less acidic than oxygenated hemoglobin and therefore ideally suited to buffer the H^+ ions (coming from tissue CO_2) in the venous blood.

6.24.) <u>OXYGEN BINDING CURVE</u>

right shift	= reduced binding of O_2
	increased protons (low pH) increased CO_2 increased 2,3-DPG increased temperature
left shift	= tighter binding of O_2
	fetal hemoglobin myoglobin

	arterial	venous
PO_2	95 mmHg	40 mmHg
O_2 saturation	97 %	70 %
PCO_2	40 mmHg	45 mm Hg
pH	7.4	7.37

6.25.) <u>BLOOD PROTEINS</u>

> **serum = plasma - fibrinogen**

	functions	decreased in:
prealbumin	- thyroxine, vitamin A	
albumin	- oncotic pressure - binds hormones, drugs	- malnutrition - liver failure - pregnancy
α1 globulin	- lipoproteins - α1 antitrypsin	- α1 deficiency
α2 globulin	- haptoglobin (carries hemoglobin dimers)	- Wilson's disease
β globulin	- transferrin (carries iron)	
γ globulin	- antibodies	- agammaglobulinemia

6.26.) <u>CIRCULATION</u>

perfusion (rest) (in % of cardiac output)	kidney > brain, muscle > heart
perfusion (exercise) (in % of cardiac output)	muscle >> heart > brain > kidney
specific perfusion (rest) (in ml min^{-1} / g tissue)	kidney >> heart > brain > muscle
largest pressure	arteries
largest resistance	arterioles
largest cross-sectional area	capillaries
largest blood volume	veins

<u>Orthostasis (standing up):</u>
- systolic pressure unchanged
- diastolic pressure increased
- peripheral resistance increased
- heart rate increased

6.27.) <u>FETAL CIRCULATION</u>

foramen ovale	right atrium -> left atrium
ductus arteriosus	pulmonary artery -> aorta
ductus venosus	umbilical vein -> vena cava inf.

- Ductus arteriosus is kept open by prostaglandins.
- Lung maturation is accelerated by glucocorticoids.

Placenta receives 30-40% of fetal blood circulation.

Head and upper extremities (<u>preductal</u>) receive O₂ rich blood.
Lower extremities (<u>postductal</u>) receive mixed blood.

6.28.) <u>RENAL TRANSPORT</u>

proximal tubule	- active resorption
	  (glucose, amino acids etc.)
	
	- active secretion
	  (organic acids, protons etc.)
	
	- carbonic anhydrase inhibitors

Henle loop	- NaCl resorption - water impermeable! (generates osmotic gradient) *- loop diuretics*
distal tubule	- K^+ secretion, H^+ secretion (in exchange for Na^+) *- thiazide diuretics*

collecting duct	- water permeable
	  (ADH increases permeability
	           -> water reabsorption)

<u>EXCRETION OF H^+ (proximal and distal tubule):</u>
- **Titratable acids:** H^+ (<1%), uric acid (10%), phosphate (40%)
- **Non-titratable acids**: NH_4^+ (50%)

<u>RECOVERY OF BICARBONATE (proximal tubule):</u>
- 99.9% of filtered HCO_3^- is recovered.
- H^+ is secreted (in exchange for Na^+) and combines with tubular HCO_3^- forming H_2CO_3 which dissociated into H_2O and CO_2. CO_2 diffuses into the cell and is split back into H^+ for secretion and HCO_3^- which then is transported through the basolateral membrane (carrier mediated) into the peritubular space.

6.29.) <u>CLEARANCE</u>

	normal value	calculated from measurement of:
RBF (renal blood flow)	1,200 mL / min	PAH clearance and hematocrit
RPF (renal plasma flow)	600 mL / min	PAH clearance
GFR (glomerular filtration rate)	125 mL / min	inulin clearance or creatinine clearance
FF (filtration fraction)	20 %	GFR / RPF

clearance > GFR	filtration + net secretion
clearance = GFR	filtration only (or secretion = resorption)
clearance < GFR	filtration + net resorption

- *Contraction of afferent arteriole decreases GFR.*
- *Contraction of efferent arteriole increases GFR.*

6.30.) <u>VOLUME REGULATION</u>

	receptors	mechanism
osmoregulation	- hypothalamus	hyperosmolarity results in: - thirst - ADH release
volume regulation	- baroreceptors - macula densa	blood volume loss results in: - sympathetic activation - renin release from JGA

	ICV	ECV	
hypotone dehydration	↑	↓	- diarrhea, vomiting
isotone dehydration	Ø	↓	- blood loss
hypertone dehydration	↓	↓	- excessive sweating - diabetes insipidus
hypotone hydration	↑	↑	- SIADH
isotone hydration	Ø	↑	- cardiac failure - nephrotic syndrome
hypertone hydration	↓	↑	- hyperaldosteronism

6.31.) <u>RENIN / ANGIOTENSIN</u>

	produced by:	features:
angiotensinogen	liver	α2 globulin
((renin))	kidney (JGA)	protease
angiotensin I		
((converting enzyme))	lung	protease
angiotensin II		vasoconstriction
aldosterone	zona glomerulosa	Na^+ reabsorption K^+ secretion
atrial natriuretic peptide (ANP)	heart: stretch of atria (high ECV)	natriuresis
natriuretic factor (ouabain-like inhibitor of Na^+/K^+ pump)		unknown significance

---

JG cells are epithelioid cells of the afferent arteriole
Macula densa is modified epithelium of distal tubule, juxtaglomerular.

Renin is released when : blood pressure at JG cells is low.
NaCl delivery to macula densa is low.

Patients with Bartter's syndrome :
high renin, angiotensin and aldosterone, but normotensive!
(down regulation of vascular angiotensin receptors?)

Patients with hypertension respond to ACE inhibitors even when their
renin levels are normal or low!

6.32.) <u>INTESTINAL ABSORPTION</u>

carbohydrates	duodenum	jejunum	
amino acids	duodenum	jejunum	
iron	duodenum		
vit. B12			terminal ileum
bile salts			terminal ileum

<u>*Iron:*</u>
- *absorbed as Fe^{2+} (combine with anti-oxidants like vit. C)*
- *transported as transferrin*
- *stored as ferritin and hemosiderin*

<u>*Defects of amino acid transporters:*</u>
Hartnup disease : defect in neutral amino acid transporter
Cystinuria :   defect in basic amino acid transporter

6.33.) <u>STOMACH</u>

	mainly secretes:
chief cells [1]	- pepsinogen
parietal cells [1]	- HCl - intrinsic factor
mucus cells [1,2]	- mucus
G cells (antrum) [2]	- gastrin

[1] fundus and corpus   [2] antrum

6.34.) <u>GI HORMONES</u>

	released by:	results in:
gastrin	- vagus (ACh) - peptides, alcohol and alkaline pH in stomach	- HCl secretion - increased stomach motility - delayed stomach emptying
secretin	- acidic pH in duodenum	- HCO_3^- rich pancreatic secretion
CCK	- fat and peptides in duodenum	- enzyme rich pancreatic secretion - gallbladder contractions
GIP	- glucose, fat in duodenum	- stimulates insulin secretion
somatostatin	- acidic pH in stomach	- inhibits HCl secretion (stomach) - inhibits enzyme secretion (pancreas)

6.35.) ADRENAL HORMONES

	released by:	syndromes
aldosterone	- basal secretion! - Angiotensin II - high [K$^+$] (ACTH)	<u>**Conn**</u> (hyper...) - K$^+$ depletion - hypertension - but not edematous ! - not hypernatremic ! - weakness, tetany <u>**Addison**</u> (hypo...) - Na$^+$ loss (hypotension) - K$^+$ retention - H$^+$ retention (metabolic acidosis) - pigmentation
cortisol	- stress - ACTH	<u>**Cushing**</u> (hyper...) - skin atrophy - muscle wasting - moon face - decreased glucose tolerance - poor wound healing - osteoporosis

Most adrenalectomized patients could survive on mineralocorticoids alone, but would face potentially fatal hypoglycemic episodes.

6.36.) INSULIN

	liver	muscle	fat cells
carbohydrates	glycogen synthesis↑ gluconeogenesis↓	glucose transport↑ glycolysis↑ glycogen synthesis↑	glucose transport↑ glycerol synthesis↑
proteins		amino acid uptake↑ protein synthesis↑	
fat	lipogenesis↑		triglyceride synthesis↑ lipolysis↓

Insulin receptor: α subunit binds insulin
β subunit has tyrosine kinase activity:
- phosphorylates itself (autophosphorylation)
- phosphorylates many other proteins
- activates ras -> raf -> MAP kinase cascade

6.37.) GONADOTROPE HORMONES

	ovaries	testes
FSH	follicle maturation	spermatogenesis
LH = ICSH	triggers ovulation luteinization of follicle	testosterone secretion (Leydig cells)

SOCIAL SCIENCE

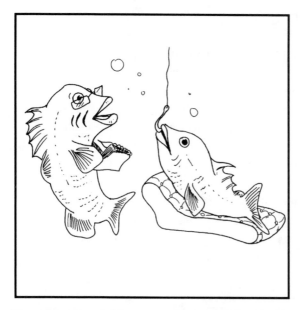

"And how long have you been feeling that
people are after you?"

Part A : Psychology

7.1.) <u>MOTOR DEVELOPMENT</u>

chin up	1 month
chest up	2 month
knee push and "swim"	6 month
sits alone / stands with help	7 month
crawls on stomach	8 month
stands holding on furniture	10 month
walks when led	11 month
stands alone	14 month
walks alone	15 month

<u>AT THE PLAYGROUND</u>:
- **stranger anxiety:**   0~1 years
- **separation anxiety:**   1~3 years
- **parallel play:**   2~3 years
- **group play:**   3~4 years

7.2.) PSYCHOLOGICAL DEVELOPMENT

years	Erikson	Freud	Piaget
0 - 1.5	trust vs. mistrust	oral (trust & dependence)	sensorimotor
1.5 - 3	autonomy vs. shame	anal (holding vs. letting out)	preoperational
3 - 6	initiative vs. guilt	phallic (Oedipus complex)	"
6 - 11	industry vs. inferiority	latency	concrete operational
11 - 20	identity vs. role confusion	genital	formal operational
20 - 25	intimacy vs. isolation		
25 - 50	generativity vs. stagnation		
50 - ?	integrity vs. despair		

7.3.) <u>IQ TESTS</u>

Deviation Tests	Tests of Mental Age
mean: 100 **standard deviation: 15** normed for each age group	IQ = mental age / biological age
WAIS adults **WISC** children **WPPSI** preschool	**Stanford Binet** (for children 3-12 years)

<u>Degrees of Mental Retardation</u>

IQ 55 - 70 (mild)	mentally handicapped educable
IQ 40 - 55 (moderate)	trainable for personal hygiene
IQ 25 - 40 (severe)	custodial
IQ < 25 (profound)	custodial

7.4.) <u>CONDITIONING</u>

"classical"	"operant"
unconditioned stimulus: meat **unconditioned response**: salivation	**operant** : behavior to be modified
conditioned stimulus: bell **conditioned response**: salivation	**positive reinforcer**: candy **negative reinforcer**: shock **primary reward** : food, sex **secondary reward** : money, praise
works on reflexive behavior (autonomic nervous system)	works on autonomic nervous system or complex behavior
reinforcement (unconditioned stimulus) occurs regardless of response	reward / punishment depend on response
partial reinforcement hastens extinction	partial or variable reinforcement results in greater resistance to extinction (examples: fishing, gambling addiction…)

 Extinction: *Disappearance of learned behavior*

7.5.) <u>DEFENSE MECHANISMS</u>

- **Regression**
  Returning to immature ways of dealing with stress: crying, tantrums…

- **Repression**
  Blocking of unacceptable urges and feelings from awareness.

- **Denial**
  Blocking of unacceptable information or perceptions from awareness.

- **Rationalization**
  Substituting an acceptable motive for attitudes or behavior for an unacceptable motive.

- **Splitting**
  Maintaining a perception of others (or self) as all good or all bad.

- **Projection**
  "You are acting like a teenager, not I !"

- **Reaction formation**
  You want to 'kick his ass' but end up kissing it...

- **Isolation of affect**
  She talked about her child's death calmly, without a sad expression in her face.

- **Displacement**
  You are angry with your boss and shout at your kids and husband instead.

- **Undoing**
  "Magic": knocking on wood etc.

Transference
Unconscious tendency of patient to respond to the therapist as if he/she were someone else.

Countertransference
Unconscious tendency of therapist to respond to the patient as if he/she were someone else.

7.6.) <u>SLEEP STAGES</u>

	key features	EEG
awake		beta: <12 / min alpha: 8-12 / min
stage 1		theta: 4-8 / min
stage 2		low voltage sleep spindles
stages 3 and 4	- night terrors - sleep walking - sleep talking - (enuresis)	delta: 1-4 / min

REM	- rapid eye movements
	- paralysis of skeletal muscles
	  (except eyes, finger, toes)
	- increased blood pressure
	  respiration
	- penis erection
	- dreams, nightmares
		like awake state

Night terrors: extreme fright, no memory or dream

Narcolepsy: - patient suddenly falls asleep (REM at onset!)
- cataplexy (sudden collapse because of loss of muscle tone)
- hypnagogic hallucinations (just before falling asleep)
- sleep paralysis (awake but unable to move or speak)

Sleep apnea: <u>*central*</u>*: no respiratory effort*
<u>*obstructive*</u>*: increased respiratory effort against*
airway obstruction

7.7.) <u>SUICIDE</u>

<u>Risk factors:</u> - has specific plan (always ask!)
- lack of social support
- recovery phase of depression
- physicians, dentists

- success-rate: 10%
- after failed attempts: 30% will try again
- 80% have given warning

- **women:** more overall attempt than men
- **men:** more "successful" suicides than women
- more common in **elderly**
- more common in **single** than in married people
- more common in **divorced** than in single people

<u>LEADING CAUSES OF DEATH:</u>

White teenagers: motor vehicle accidents > suicides > homicides
Black teenagers: homicides > motor vehicle accidents > suicides

7.8.) <u>STAGES OF DYING</u>
Elisabeth Kübler-Ross

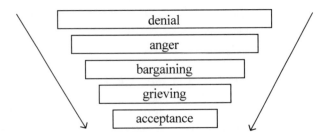

Part B : Psychopathology

7.9.) <u>NEUROTRANSMTTERS</u>

schizophrenia	dopamine
depression	norepinephrine serotonin dopamine
Alzheimer's disease	acetylcholine
anxiety	GABA

Benzodiazepines and barbiturates act on GABA receptors:
-> open Cl⁻ channels
-> hyperpolarization of nerve cell
-> decreased neuronal firing

7.10.) <u>GRIEF & DEPRESSION</u>

grief	depression
- initial: shock/denial - illusions / hallucinations may occur - low risk of suicide	- feeling of hopelessness - feeling of worthlessness - high risk of suicide

<u>Abnormal grief reaction:</u>
- *continued thoughts about guilt and death*
- *marked psychomotor retardation*
- *marked functional impairment*
- *lasts < 2 months (if longer, a diagnosis of major depression is likely)*

7.11.) <u>DELIRIUM & DEMENTIA</u>

delirium	dementia
- impaired consciousness (agitation or stupor)	- unimpaired consciousness
- develops quickly - usually reversible	- develops slowly - irreversible

7.12.) <u>PERSONALITY TYPES</u>

Patients usually are not distressed about their personality type.

dependent	afraid of being helpless need to be cared for
compulsive	fear of loss of control tries to control physician
passive-aggressive	appears willing but is non-compliant
histrionic	dramatic, emotional may display inappropriate sexual behavior
narcissistic	feels better than others perfect self-image is threatened by disease
paranoid	may blame physician or others for disease
schizoid	anxious, withdrawn (doesn't want close relationships)

Personality disorder: *Inflexible pattern, significant deviation from cultural norm, significant distress or functional impairment.*

"Borderline": *Severe personality disorder with features of psychoses. Intense unstable relationships, self-damaging, suicidal behavior, paranoia, dissociations.*

7.13.) <u>ANXIETY DISORDERS</u>

Patients are distressed and know that their symptoms are irrational.

phobia	- persistent excessive of specific objects or situations - patient knows that his fear his unrealistic
agoraphobia	- history of panic attacks - patient avoids places were panic attack might occur (especially public places)
obsessive compulsive	- *obsessions*: recurrent thoughts - *compulsions*: repetitive behavior
posttraumatic stress disorder	- traumatic event in history - may occur ANY time after event - persists for > 1 month

7.14.) <u>SOMATOFORM DISORDERS</u>

somatization (Briquet's syndrome)	- sickly for most of life - GI, reproductive, cardiopulmonary, pain etc. - diagnosed, when at least 12 symptoms are present and history of several years.
conversion disorder (hysterical neurosis)	- "pseudo-neurological" (blindness, paresthesia, paralysis) - symptoms begin and end suddenly - often misdiagnosed as "malingering"
hypochondriasis	- unrealistic interpretation of body signs - belief to have serious disease that goes unrecognized by family and physicians

7.15.) <u>PSYCHOSES</u>

schizophrenia	<u>**positive symptoms:**</u> - delusions - hallucinations (often auditory) <u>**negative symptoms:**</u> - flat affect - avolition <u>**"four A's":**</u> - affect inappropriate - ambivalence - associative thinking (alogical) - autism
major depression	- depressed mood - feeling of worthlessness - weight loss - early morning insomnia
bipolar type 1	- at least <u>one manic</u> episode in patient's history
bipolar type 2	- at least <u>one major depressive</u> episode PLUS - at least <u>one hypomanic episode</u>

 You should NOT make diagnosis of major depression within two months after bereavement (loss of a loved-one), even if the "classical" symptoms are present!

7.16.) <u>EPILEPSY</u>

grand mal	- tonic, then clonic - loss of consciousness - incontinence - EEG : high voltage spikes
petit mal	- absence seizure ("blank spell") - no loss of muscle tone - EEG : 3/sec spikes and domes
narcolepsy	- loss of muscle tone - REM onset sleep
psychomotor	- non-goal directed activity (lip smacking, walking...) - EEG : spikes in temporal lobes
Jacksonian	- spreading muscle group activity (e.g. fingers -> forearm -> shoulder) - EEG : focus around antral sulcus

7.17.) <u>DRUG ABUSE</u>

Abuse:	Recurrent use of drugs resulting in social failures (at home, school or work), legal problems or hazardous situations.
Dependence:	Tolerance (needs larger doses to achieve effect). Withdrawal symptoms.

	intoxication	withdrawal
alcohol	- euphoria - disorientation - unsteady gait	- nausea - tremor, seizures - delusions, hallucinations - delirium tremens
barbiturates	- sedation	- can be severe! - delirium - epilepsy - coma, death
benzodiazepines	- antianxiety - sedation	- anxiety - irritability - insomnia
amphetamines, cocaine	- arousal - euphoria	- fatigue - dysphoria
opioids	- euphoria - apathy	- nausea, vomiting - sweating, fever - muscle ache
LSD	- hallucinations - anxiety - paranoid ideas	none

Blood alcohol: *>100 mg/dL → intoxication*
>200 mg/dL → fall asleep, anesthesia
>400 mg/dL → inhibition of respiration, death

Metabolic rate is 15-20 mg/dL per hour

7.18.) CHILD ABUSE

physical	sexual
infants, younger children	preadolescent, adolescents
abuser often female	abuser usually male abuser usually known to victim
RISK FACTORS: - prematurity, low birth weight - drug abuse - parents abused as children - poverty	RISK FACTORS: - drug abuse - single-parent home

perhaps accidental	more likely intentional
• splash marks • injuries to front • foot soles spared	• clearly demarcated areas, no splash • injuries to back • foot soles involved • history of multiple injuries • retinal hemorrhage ("shaken baby")

Part C : Statistics

7.19.) <u>DEFINITIONS</u>

- **Standard deviation**: ±1s includes 68%, ±2s includes 95%, ±3s includes 99%

- **Mean**: average value
  Median: half the values are higher, half the values are lower than this
  Mode: most common value
  In a perfectly symmetrical non-skewed distribution, mean, median and mode are the same.

- **Relative risk:** (incidence with risk factor) / (incidence without risk factor)
- **Attributable risk:** (incidence with risk factor) - (incidence without risk factor)

- **Chi square test.** Analysis of categorical data distribution.
  Example: Two groups of patients with chronic arthritis are given either drug or placebo. Condition after treatment will be rated "improved", "same", or "worsened".

- **Paired Student's t-test.** Each patient serves as its own control.
  Example: A group of patients with hypertension is treated first with placebo then with drug (or vice versa) in a "cross-over" design.

- **Correlation coefficient.** Test of degree of association between two variables.
  Blood pressure and triglyceride levels are measured in a cross-sectional study of patients.

- **Analysis of variance.** Determine how several independent variables affect one dependent variable (similar to t-test, but more variables).
  Example: Effect of blood pressure, cholesterol, triglycerides and patient's income on incidence of myocardial infarction.

- **Analysis of covariance.** Determine how several independent variables affect one dependent variable and controlling for other variables.
  Example: Assessment of effect of drug versus placebo in two groups of patients taking pretreatment blood pressure into account.

320

7.20.) <u>SENSITIVITY</u>

	patient is sick	patient is healthy
test result is positive	A	B
test result is negative	C	D

Sensitivity: divide A by (A+C)
C = "False negative"

Definition:
Sensitivity is the probability that a sick patient (A+C) will have a positive test result (A).

- Tests with high sensitivity are used for screening.
- Tests with high sensitivity are used to "rule out" diagnosis.

"A test has a sensitivity of 90%" means that 10% of patients with the disease go undetected (C = false negative).

7.21.) <u>SPECIFICITY</u>

	patient is sick	patient is healthy
test result is positive	A	B
test result is negative	C	D

Specificity: divide D by (B+D)
B = "False positive"

Definition:
Specificity is the probability that a healthy patient (B+D)
will have a negative test result (D).

- Tests with high specificity are used for confirmation.
- Tests with high sensitivity are used to "rule in" diagnosis.

---

*"A test has a specificity" of 80% means that 20% of people
without disease get a false positive (B) test result.*

*Sensitivity and specificity are independent of disease
prevalence!*

7.22.) <u>POSITIVE PREDICTIVE VALUE</u>

	patient is sick	patient is healthy
test result is positive	(A)	B
test result is negative	C	D

Positive predictive value: divide A by (A+B)

<hr>

Definition:
PPV is the probability that a patient with a positive test result (A+B) is indeed sick (A).

<hr>

The predictive value depends not only on the test's properties but also on disease prevalence.

For example, if you had screened inhabitants of Siberia in 1985 for HIV antibodies, all positive results would have been false positive and the PPV would have been 0.

Similarly, screening an asymptomatic, low-risk population will result in many false positives. The expense for follow-up of false positive results (plus the alarm you cause the patient) needs to be weighed against the benefits of early disease detection.

7.23.) <u>NEGATIVE PREDICTIVE VALUE</u>

	patient is sick	patient is healthy
test result is positive	A	B
test result is negative	C	D

Negative predictive value: divide D by (C+D)

Definition:
NPV is the probability that a patient with a negative test
result (C+D) is indeed healthy (D).

PPV is higher in populations with high prevalence!
NPV is higher in populations with low prevalence!

7.24.) <u>CANCER STATISTICS (USA)</u>

A.) <u>Incidence</u>
  - *number of <u>new</u> people that develop disease*
  - *in one year per 100,000 population*

Male	female
1. prostate (41%)	1. breast (31%)
2. lung (13%)	2. lung (13%)
3. colorectal (9%)	3. colorectal (11%)

B.) <u>Mortality</u>
  - *number of people who die of disease*
  - *in one year per 100,000 population*

male	female
1. lung (32%)	1. lung (25%)
2. prostate (14%)	2. breast (17%)
3. colorectal (9%)	3. colon (10%)

C.) <u>Prevalence</u>
  - *number of people who have disease*
  - *at a given date (or time interval) per 100,000 population*
  - *depends on both incidence and duration of disease!*

7.25.) <u>RANDOMIZED CLINICAL TRIAL</u>

"State of the Art" test to evaluate new drugs

design	researcher conducts interventions
study group	patients are selected and assigned randomly to intervention or control groups
observation	patients are assessed before and after intervention or control procedure

Null hypothesis: assumes that there is no significant difference (between new drug and control treatment)

Type I error: null hypothesis is rejected although it is true

Type II error: null hypothesis is not rejected even though it is false

p value: probability of a type I error

The lower the p value the better.
(high probability that there indeed is a significant difference)

7.26.) <u>OBSERVATIONAL COHORT</u>
(prospective)

design	researcher observes natural events over time (no intervention, requires lots of time and effort)
study group	two patient groups defined by presence/absence of risk factors are compared
observation	patients are assessed repeatedly during course of study <u>to estimate incidence of disease in groups with different risk factors</u>

Validity: does the test measure what it is supposed to measure?
Reliability: how well can the test results be reproduced?

<u>Framingham Heart Study:</u>
- sample population of Framingham, Massachusetts
- assesses risk factors for cardiovascular disease
- began in 1950, still ongoing today

7.27.) <u>CASE CONTROL STUDY</u>
(retrospective)

design	researcher determines presence of risk factors retrospectively
study group	two patient groups defined by presence/absence of disease are compared
observation	patients are assessed for presence of disease at begin of study, then questioned for risk factors

7.28.) <u>CROSS SECTIONAL SURVEY</u>
(convenient, common study)

design	researcher records presence of variables (can be done on existing data base)
study group	single patient group for which association between variables is sought
observation	data are obtained on all variables of interest at the same point of time <u>to determine if there is a correlation of two or more variables</u>

Correlation coefficient: +1   *perfect correlation*
                      0   *no correlation between variables*
                     -1   *perfect negative correlation*

7.29.) <u>LEGAL ISSUES</u>

- Competent patients may refuse medical treatment, even if death will result.

- **Involuntary treatment** requires a) patient is mentally ill
  PLUS
  b) danger to self or others

- **Living will**: Directions for future care (when unable to make decisions)
- **Durable power of attorney**: designate a legal representative to make decisions

- **Confidentiality**: May be breached if significant risk to others exists:
  (HIV positive prostitute, patient threatens to kill, child abuse)

- **Minors**: Parents must give consent
- No consent necessary if: - emergency
  - pregnancy
  - treatment of sexually transmitted diseases

- Some States require parental consent for abortion, others do not.

- Self-supporting minors are considered adults. Parental consent is not necessary

- **Medicare**: Care for the elderly (>65 years, part of "Social Security")
- **Medicaid**: Aid for the poor (on welfare)

- **HMOs** - prepaid insurance plan
  - physicians are paid fixed salary to take care of group of people

ABBREVIATIONS

a/w	associated with	LSD	lysergic acid diethylamide
AA	amyloid associated protein	MAC	minimal alveolar concentration
Ab	antibodies	MAO	monoamine oxidase
ACh	acetylcholine	MHC	major histocompatibility complex
ADHD	attention deficit hyperactivity disorder	MI	myocardial infarction
AFP	alpha fetoprotein	MIF	Müllerian inhibiting factor
AL	amyloid light chains	MLC	myosin light chain
ALA	aminolevulinic acid	MODY	maturity onset diabetes of the young
ANA	antinuclear antibodies	MS	multiple sclerosis
AP	action potential	NIDDM	non insulin dependent diabetes mellitus
aPTT	partial thromboplastin time	NSAID	nonsteroidal antiinflammatory drug
ASD	atrial septal defect	PAH	p-aminohippurate
ARDS	acute respiratory distress syndrome	PAS	periodic acid Schiff reagent
BP	blood pressure	PCP	phencyclidine
CA	carcinoma	PDA	patent ductus arteriosus
CEA	carcinoembryonic antigen	PDE	phosphodiesterase
CoA	coenzyme A	PG	prostaglandin
COPD	chronic obstructive pulmonary disease	PMN	polymorph nuclear leukocyte
CSF	cerebrospinal fluid	PT	prothrombin time
CNS	central nervous system	RBC	red blood cells
DES	diethylstilbestrol	RSV	respiratory syncytial virus
DIC	disseminated intravascular coagulation	SLE	systemic lupus erythematosus
DOC	drug of choice	ss	single stranded
ds	double stranded	SSPE	subacute sclerosing panencephalitis
DX	differential diagnosis	TCA	tricyclic antidepressants
EBV	Epstein-Barr virus	THC	tetrahydrocannabinol
ECV	extracellular volume	TIA	transient ischemic attack
EEE	eastern equine encephalitis	TPA	tissue plasminogen activator
G6PD	glucose-6-phosphate dehydrogenase	TRAP	tartrate resistant alkaline phosphatase
GABA	gamma-aminobutyrate	TT	thrombin time
GBM	glomerular basement membrane	TX	treatment
GH	growth hormone	UMN	upper motor neuron
GI	gastrointestinal	UTI	urinary tract infection
GN	glomerulonephritis	VD	venereal disease
HCG	human chorionic gonadotropin	VDRL	Venereal Disease Research Laboratory
!DDM	insulin dependent diabetes mellitus	VSD	ventricular septal defect
JGA	juxtaglomerular apparatus	VZV	varicella zoster virus
LMN	lower motor neuron	WEE	western equine encephalitis

INDEX

11-β-hydroxylase deficiency, **4.38**
17-α-hydroxylase deficiency, **4.36**
17-hydroxysteroids, 4.28
17-ketosteroids, 4.28
21-α-hydroxylase deficiency, **4.37**
5th disease, 2.22
6th disease, 2.23
Abdominal arteries, **5.20**
Abducens paralysis, 5.7
Abnormal grief reaction, 7.10
Accommodation, 5.7, **6.7**
ACE inhibitors, 3.19
Acetaminophen, 3.17, 3.4
Acetazolamide, 3.22
Achondroplasia, 1.13, 1.72
Acid phosphatase, 1.9
Acid/base, 6.1, **6.22**
Acidosis, 6.22
Actinic keratosis, 1.87
Actinomyces, 2.18, 3.6
Actinomycin D, 3.14, 3.15
Acute intermittent porphyria, 4.20
Acute renal failure, 1.17
Acyclovir, 3.9
Addison's disease, 6.35
Adenovirus, 2.22
ADHD, 3.44
Adrenal adenoma, **1.81**
Adrenal gland, **4.29**
Adrenal hormones, **6.35**
Adrenergic drugs, **3.34**
Adrenergic receptors, **6.13**
Adrenoleukodystrophy, 1.78
Aerobe, 2.5
AFP, 1.51
Agoraphobia, 7.13
AIDS, **3.12**.
Albinism, 1.12, 4.4, 4.5
Albumin, 6.25
Albuterol, 3.28, 3.34

Alcohol abuse, 7.17
Aldosterone, 6.35
Alkaline phosphatase, 1.9
Alkalosis, 6.22
Alkaptonuria, 4.4, 4.5
ALL, 1.28, 3.16
Allantois, 5.5
Allopurinol, 3.18
All-or-none response, 6.5
Alpha1-antitrypsin deficiency, 1.12
Alpha-agonists, 3.34
Alpha-amanitin, 1.89, 3.15
Alpha-blockers, 3.34
Alpha-fetoprotein, 1.9
Alpha-receptors, 6.13
Alpha-toxin, 2.4, 2.7
Aluminum, 3.33
Alveolar proteinosis, 1.44
Alzheimer's disease, 1.77
Amanitin, 3.15
Amantadine, 3.9, 3.49
Amebiasis, 3.11
Amenorrhea, 1.17
Amiloride, 3.22
Amino acid disorders, **4.4**
Amino acid precursors, **4.3**
Amino acids, **4.2**
Aminoglycosides, **3.2**, 3.13
Amiodarone, 3.26
Amitriptyline, 3.42
AML, 1.28
Amoxapine, 3.42
Amphetamine, 3.34, 3.44, 7.17
Amphotericin, 3.10
Ampicillin, 3.7
Amrinone, 3.27
Amyloid, **1.5**
Amyotrophic lateral sclerosis, 1.77, 5.35
Anabolic, 4.39
Anaerobe, 2.5

Anaphylactic shock, 3.3
Anemia, 1.17, **1.24**
Anesthetics, **3.48**
Aneurysms, **1.34**
Angelman syndrome, 1.15
Angina, 1.37, 3.23
Angiotensin, **6.31**
Angiotensin antagonists, **3.20**
Ankle, **5.17**
Ankle jerk reflex, 5.37
Ankylosing spondylitis, 1.16
Anomers, 4.6
Antacids, 3.33
Anthrax, 2.11, 3.6
Antianginal drugs, **3.23**
Antiarrhythmic drugs, **3.26**
Antibiotics, **3.5**
Anticoagulants, **3.25**
Antidepressants, **3.42**
Antidotes, **3.4**
Antiemetic drugs, **3.52**
Antiepileptic drugs, **3.51**
Anti-folates, 3.14
Antifungal drugs, **3.10**
Antigenic drift, 2.24
Antigenic shift, 2.24
Antihistamines, **3.47**
Antihypertensive drugs, **3.19**
Antiprotozoal drugs, **3.11**
Antiviral drugs, **3.9**
Anxiety disorders, **7.13**
Anxiolytic drugs, **3.45**
Aortic regurgitation, 1.35
Aortic stenosis, 1.35
Aphasias, 5.24
Aplastic anemia, 1.24
Appendicitis, 5.21
Arachidonic acid, 4.14
ARBO viruses, **2.25**
ARDS, 1.44
Arsenic, 1.89
Arteriosclerosis, **1.32**
Arteritis, **1.33**
Arthritis, **1.71**

Arthus reaction, 1.6
Asbestos, 1.89
Ascaris, 2.37
Aschoff body, 1.42
Aseptic necrosis, 1.72
Aspergillosis, 2.31
Aspirin, 3.17, 3.24, 6.22
Astemizole, 3.47
Asthma, 1.43, **3.28**
Astrocytoma, 1.76
Atenolol, 3.34
Atherosclerosis, 1.32
Atonic bladder, 3.36
ATP equivalents, 4.24
Atrial natriuretic peptide, 6.31
Atrial septal defect, 1.36
Atropine, 3.37
Atypical pneumonia, 1.45, 3.6
Auditory meatus, 5.6
Autoantibodies, **1.4**
Automatic bladder, 3.36
Autonomic nervous system, **6.11**
Autosomal dominant diseases, **1.13**
Autosomal recessive diseases, **1.12**
Azathioprine, 3.14
AZT, 3.9, 3.12, 4.40
Bacilli, **2.10**
Bacillus anthracis, 2.11
Bactericidal, 3.5
Bacteriostatic, 3.5
Bacteroides fragilis, 2.14
Barbiturates, 3.46, 7.9, 7.17
Basal cell carcinoma, 1.87
Basal ganglia, **5.30**
Basilar skull fractures, 5.6
Basophil stippling, 1.25
Becker's dystrophy, 1.14, 1.75
Bence-Jones protein, 1.30
Benzene, 1.89
Benzodiazepines, 3.4, 3.45, 7.9, 7.17
Benztropine, 3.49
Berger's disease, 1.47
Berry aneurysms, 1.13
Beta-agonists, 3.27, 3.34

Beta-blockers, 3.19, 3.34
Beta-lactamase, 3.7
Beta-receptors, 6.13
Bethanechol, 3.36
Bicarbonate, 6.1, 6.28
Bile acids, **4.15**
Biot respiration, 6.20
Biperiden, 3.49
Bipolar disorder, 7.15
Bismuth, 3.33
Bladder, urinary, 3.36
Blastomycosis, 2.31
Bleeding disorders, **1.22**
Bleomycin, 3.14, 3.16
Blood alcohol, 7.17
Blood pressure, 6.11
Blood proteins, **6.25**
Bone diseases, **1.72**
Bone marrow suppression, 3.3
Bone tumors, **1.74**
Borderline personality, 7.12
Bordetella, 2.16
Bornholm disease, 2.24
Borrelia burgdorferi, 2.19
Botulinum toxin, 2.4
Botulism, 2.12
Bovine spongiform encephalopathy, 2.27
Bowen's disease, 1.87
Brachial plexus, **5.12**, **5.13**
Brain tumors, **1.76**
Brainstem syndromes, **5.32 - 5.35**
Branchial arches, **5.3**
Breast diseases, **1.55**
Breathing patterns, **6.20**
Bretylium, 3.26
Briquet's syndrome, 7.14
Broca, 5.24
Bromocriptine, 3.21, 3.49
Bronchiectasis, 1.43
Bronchitis, 1.43, 2.6
Bronchopneumonia, 1.45
Brucella, 2.15
Bruton's agammaglobulinemia, 1.14, 1.21
Burkitt lymphoma, 1.7, 1.29, 2.23

Buspirone, 3.45
Butyrophenone, 3.50
C. donovani, 1.50
Cadmium, 1.89
Caffeine, 3.44
Calcium channel blockers, 3.19
cAMP, 6.4
Campylobacter jejuni, 2.14, 3.6
Cancer statistics, **7.24**
Candida, 1.50, 2.31, 3.6, 3.10, 3.12
Captopril, 3.20
Carbachol, 3.36
Carbamazepine, 3.51
Carbenicillin, 3.7
Carbidopa, 3.49
Carbinoxamine, 3.47
Carbon monoxide, 3.4
Carbonic anhydrase inhibitors, 3.22
Carcinoid, 1.46
Cardiac cycle, **6.18**
Cardiac index, 6.1
Cardiac output, 6.1
Cardiolipin, 4.16
Carpal tunnel syndrome, 5.13
Cartilage, **1.73**
Case control studies, **7.27**
Castor oil, 3.53
Cat bites, 2.15
Catabolic, 4.39
Cataplexy, 7.6
Cauda equina lesion, 5.35
CCK, 6.34
CEA, 1.9
Cefamandole, 3.8
Cefazolin, 3.8
Cefotaxime, 3.8
Cefoxitin, 3.8
Ceftriaxone, 3.8
Celiac sprue, 1.4, 1.62
Celiac trunk, 5.20
Cell capsule, 2.3
Cell walls, **2.3**
Cellulose, 4.8
Cephalexin, 3.8
Cephalosporins, **3.8**

Cerebellum, 5.27
Cerebral arteries, **5.25**
Cervical cysts, 5.4
Cervix carcinoma, 2.22
Cestodes, **2.36**
Chagas disease, 3.11
Chancre, 1.50
Chancroid, 1.50
Charcot's triad, 1.63
Chédiak-Higashi syndrome, 1.12
Cheilosis, 1.56
Chemotaxis, 1.1
Chemotherapy, **3.16**
Cheyne-Stokes respiration, 6.20
Chi square test, 7.19
Chickenpox, 2.23
Chief cells, 6.33
Child abuse, **7.18**
Chlamydia, **2.20**
Chlamydia pneumoniae, 2.20
Chlamydia psittaci, 2.20
Chlamydia trachomatis, 1.50, 2.20
Chloral hydrate, 3.46
Chloramphenicol, 3.13
Chlordiazepoxide, 3.45
Chloroquine, 3.11
Chlorothiazide, 3.22
Chlorpromazine, 3.50
Chlorpropamide, 3.30
Chlorthalidone, 3.22
Cholangiocarcinoma, 1.70
Cholangitis, 1.63
Cholelithiasis, **1.63**
Cholera, 3.6
Cholera toxin, 2.4
Cholesterol, 1.13, 3.31
Cholestyramine, 3.32
Cholic acid, 4.15
Cholinergic drugs, **3.36**
Cholinesterase inhibitors, **3.35**
Chondroblastoma, 1.73
Chondrosarcoma, 1.73
Choriocarcinoma, 1.52, 1.54
Chorionic gonadotropin, 1.51

Chromium, 1.89
Chronic bronchitis, 1.43
Chronic granulomatous disease, 1.14
Chronic pancreatitis, 1.17, 1.85
Chymotrypsin, 4.2
Cimetidine, 3.33
Circulation, **6.26**
Cirrhosis, 1.68, **1.69**
Cisplatin, 3.16
Cistron, 4.44
Classical conditioning, 7.4
Clearance, 6.1, **6.29**
CLL, 1.28
Clofibrate, 3.32
Clonazepam, 3.51
Clonidine, 3.34
Clonorchis sinensis, 2.35
Clostridia, 2.11, **2.12**
Clostridium botulinum, 2.12
Clostridium perfringens, 2.12
Clostridium tetani, 2.12
Clozapine, 3.40
CML, 1.28, 1.7
CMV, 2.23, 3.12
CNS Degeneration, **1.77**
CNS stimulants, **3.44**
CO, 3.4
Cobalt, 1.89
Cocaine, 3.44, 7.17
Coccidioidomycosis, 2.31
Cochlea, **6.9**
Codeine, 3.41
Codman's triangle, 1.74
Colchicine, 3.18
Cold antibodies, 1.23
Colestipol, 3.32
Colles' fracture, 5.14
Colon carcinoma, 1.7
Colorado tick fever, 2.25
Common causes, **1.17, 2.6**
Common cold, 2.6
Complement, **1.3**
Compliance, lung, 6.1
Compulsive personality, 7.12
Conditioning, **7.4**

Condyloma acuminatum, 1.50
Confidentiality, 7.29
Congenital heart defects, **1.36**
Congo red, 2.1
Conidia, 2.30
Conjugation, 3.5
Conn's syndrome, 1.81, 6.35
Conversion disorder, 7.14
Coombs test, 1.23
COPD, 1.43, 6.20
Coronary arteries, **5.19**
Corpus luteum, **4.35**
Correlation coefficient, 7.19, 7.28
Cortex, **5.24**
Corticosteroids, 3.28
Cortisol, 4.39, 6.35
Corynebacterium, 2.11
Coumarin, 3.4
Countertransference, 7.5
Coxsackie, 2.24
Cranial nerves, **5.28**
Craniopharyngioma, 1.76
CREST, 1.19, 1.4
Creutzfeldt-Jakob disease, 2.27
Cri du chat syndrome, 1.15
Crigler-Najjar, 1.65
Crohn's disease, 1.61
Cromolyn, 3.28
Cross sectional surveys, **7.28**
Croup, 2.24
Cruciate ligament, 5.16
Cryptococcosis, 2.31
Cryptococcus neoformans, 3.12
Cryptosporidium, 2.34
Cushing's syndrome, 1.81, 6.35
Cutaneous flushing, 3.3
Cyanide, 3.4
Cycloheximide, 3.13
Cyclophosphamide, 3.16
Cystic fibrosis, 1.12
Cystinuria, 4.4
Cystitis, 2.6
Cystosarcoma phyllodes, 1.55
Cytarabine, 3.14

Cytochrome P450, 3.1
Cytokines, **1.2**
De Quervain's thyroiditis, 1.82
Dead space, 6.19
Deafness, **6.10**
Death, causes of, 7.7
Decerebrate posture, 6.15
Decorticate posture, 6.15
Defense mechanisms, **7.5**
Dehydration, 6.30
Deletions, chromosome, **1.15**
Delirium, **7.11**
Dementia, **7.11**
Demyelinating diseases, **1.78**
Dengue fever, 2.25
Denial, 7.5
Dependence, 7.17
Dependent personality, 7.12
Deprenyl, 3.49
Depression, **7.10**, 7.15
Dermatomes, **5.37**
Dermatophytic Infections, 2.31, 3.10
Desipramine, 3.42
Devic's disease, 1.78
Diabetes, **1.85**
Diacylglycerol, 6.4
Diarrhea, 2.6
Diazepam, 3.45, 3.51
Dicumarol, 3.25
Diffusion capacity, 6.1
DiGeorge syndrome, 1.21
Digitoxin, 3.27
Digoxin, 3.27
Diphenhydramine, 3.47
Diphtheria, 2.11
Diphtheria toxin, 2.4, 3.13
Diphyllobothrium latum, 2.36
Dipyridamole, 3.24
Displacement, 7.5
Diuretics, **3.22**
DNA viruses, **2.22**
Dobutamine, 3.27, 3.34
Dog bites, 2.15
Dopamine, 3.27, 3.34

Doxorubicin, 3.14, 3.15, 3.16
D-penicillamine, 3.17
Dressler syndrome, 1.41
Droperidol, 3.50
Drug abuse, **7.17**
Drug induced lupus, 1.4, 3.3
Drug interactions, **3.1**
Drug withdrawal, 7.17
Drugs of choice, **3.6**
Duchenne's dystrophy, 1.14, 1.75
Ductus arteriosus, 5.2, 6.27
Ductus venosus, 5.2, 6.27
Dwarfism, 1.80
Dying, stages of, **7.8**
Dynorphin, 3.41
Dysentery, 3.6
Dysgerminoma, 1.52
Dyskinesias, **3.50**
Dystrophin, 1.75
E. coli, 2.13
EBV, 2.23
Echinococcus, 2.36
Ectoderm, 1.76, 5.1
Edinger-Westphal nucleus, 5.29
Edrophonium, 3.35
EEE, 2.25
EEG, **7.6**, 7.16
Ehlers-Danlos syndrome, 1.13
Eisenmenger reaction, 1.36
Elbow, **5.14**
Electromechanical coupling, **6.17**
Electrophoresis, **6.25**
Emphysema, 1.43
Enalapril, 3.20
Enantiomers, 4.6
Encainide, 3.26
Enchondroma, 1.73
Endocarditis, **1.40**, 2.6, 3.6
Endoderm, 5.1
Endometrium, **1.53**
Endonuclease, 4.45
Endorphins, 3.41
Endotoxins, 2.4
Enflurane, 3.48
Enhancers, 4.43

Enkephalins, 3.41
Entamoeba histolytica, 2.34
Enterobacteriaceae, **2.13**, **2.14**
Enterobius, 2.37
Enterotoxin, 2.4, 2.7
Enzyme defects, **4.5, 4.10, 4.12, 4.19, 4.21**
Enzyme kinetics, **4.1**
Eosinophilia, 1.27
Eosinophilic pneumonia, 1.44
Ephedrine, 3.34
Epigastric arteries, 5.2
Epilepsy, **7.16**
Epimers, 4.6
Epinephrine, 4.39
Equations, **6.1**
Ergot Alkaloids, **3.21**
Ergotamine, 3.21
Erikson, 7.2
Erysipelas, 3.6
Erythema infectiosum, 2.22
Erythromycin, 3.13
Esophageal diverticula, **1.57**
Estrogens, 3.39
Ethacrynic acid, 3.22
Ethosuximide, 3.51
Ethylene glycol, 3.4
Eunuchoid, 1.80
Ewing's sarcoma, 1.74
Exfoliatin, 2.7
Exonuclease, 4.45
Exotoxins, 2.4, 2.7, 2.8
Exudation, 1.1
Eye, **5.7**
Fabry disease, 1.14, 4.18
Facilitated transport, 6.3
Fallot's tetralogy, 1.36
Familial hypercholesterolemia, 1.13
Familial polyposis, 1.13, 1.60
Famotidine, 3.33
Fanconi anemia, 1.24
Farsightedness, 6.7
Fasting, 4.22
Fatty acids, **4.14**
Febrile seizures, 3.51
Felty's syndrome, 1.26, 1.71

Femur neck fractures, 5.15
Fentanyl, 3.41
Fetal alcohol syndrome, 1.36
Fetal circulation, **6.27**
Fetal hydantoin syndrome, 1.36
Fetal remnants, **5.2**
Fever, 1.1
Fibers, 3.53
Fibroadenoma, 1.55
Fibrocystic change, 1.55
Fibrosis of lung, 1.44
Filtration fraction, 6.29
Flecainide, 3.26
Flukes, **2.35**
Fluorouracil, 3.14, 4.42
Fluoxetine, 3.42
Fluphenazine, 3.50
Food poisoning, 1.17
Foramen magnum, 5.6
Foramen ovale, 5.6, 6.27
Foramen rotundum, 5.6
Foramen spinosum, 5.6
Fragile, X 1.14
Framingham heart study, 7.26
Francisella, 2.15
Frank Starling mechanism, 6.14
Freud, 7.2
Friedreich's ataxia, 1.77
Fructose intolerance, 4.9, 4.10
Fructosuria, 4.9
FSH, 6.37
Fungal diseases, **2.31**, 3.10
Fungi, **2.30**
Furanose, 4.6
Furosemide, 3.22

G proteins, **6.4**
G6PD deficiency, 1.14, 1.23, 3.3
Galactosemia, 4.9, 4.10
Gallbladder carcinoma, **1.64**
Ganciclovir, 3.9
Gardner's syndrome, 1.60
Gastric ulcer, 3.6
Gastrin, 6.34
Gastritis, **1.58**

Gastroenteritis, **1.59**
Gastrointestinal hormones, **6.34**
Gaucher's disease, 4.18
Gene expression, **4.43**
Genetics of disease, **1.11**
Genital herpes, 1.50
Germ cell tumors, 1.51
Germ layers, **5.1**
German measles, 2.24
Gestational diabetes, 1.85
Ghon complex, 2.17
Giant cell arteritis, 1.33
Giardia lamblia, 2.34
Giemsa, 2.1
Gilbert's syndrome, 1.65
GIP, 6.34
Glioblastoma, 1.76
Glipizide, 3.30
Globulin, 6.25
Glomerular filtration rate, 6.29
Glomerulonephritis, **1.47**
Glomerulonephritis, **1.48**
Glossitis, 1.56
Glucagon, 4.39
Glucogenic, 4.2
Glucokinase, **4.7**
Glyburide, 3.30
Glycerophosphate shuttle, 4.24
Glycogen, 4.8
Glycogen storage diseases, 1.12, **4.11**
Glycolipids, 4.17
Glycosaminoglycans, **4.13**
Glycosides, 3.27
Gold, 3.17
Golgi tendon organ, 6.15
Gonadotrope hormones, **6.37**
Gonococcus, 2.9
Gonorrhea, 3.6
Goodpasture syndrome, 1.4, 1.44, 1.47
Gout, **3.18**
Gower's sign, 1.75
gp120, 2.29
gp41, 2.29
Gram stain, 2.1
Gram-negative bacilli, **2.15**, **2.16**

Gram-positive bacilli, **2.11**
Grand mal, 3.51, 7.16
Granuloma inguinale, 1.50
Granulosa cells, **4.33**
Graves' disease, 1.4, 1.82
Grief, **7.10**
Griseofulvin, 3.10
Group play, 7.1
Growth hormone, 4.39
Guanethidine, 3.34
Guillain-Barré syndrome, 1.78, 5.35
H⁺, kidneys, 6.28
Hairy cell leukemia, 1.28
Hallucinogens, **3.40**
Haloperidol, 3.50
Halothane, 1.68, 3.48
Hamstrings, 5.16
Hand-foot-mouth disease, 2.24
Hantavirus, 2.25
Hartnup disease, 4.4
Hashimoto's thyroiditis, 1.4, 1.82
Heart beat, **6.14**
Heart failure, **1.39**
Heart muscle, **6.17**
Heart sounds, **1.35**
Heberden's nodes, 1.71
Heinz bodies, 1.25
Helicase, 4.45
Helicobacter pylori, 1.58, 2.14, 3.33
Hemangioblastoma, 1.76
Hemangioma, 1.88
Hematopoiesis, 1.2
Hemianopsia, 5.25
Hemochromatosis, 1.12, 1.16, 1.69, 1.85
Hemoglobin, **6.23**
Hemolytic anemias, **1.23**
Hemophilia, 1.14, 1.22
Hemophilus, 2.16
Hemophilus ducreyi, 1.50
Hemorrhage, intracranial, **5.27**
Henderson-Hasselbalch equation, 6.1
Henle loop, 6.28
Hepadnavirus, 2.22
Heparin, 3.4, 3.25

Hepatitis, **1.66**
Hepatitis serology, **1.67**
Hepatotoxicity, 3.3
Herpangina, 2.24
Herpes, 3.12
Herpes viruses, **2.23**
Heterophil negative mononucleosis, 2.23
Hexokinase, **4.7**
Hexoses, **4.6**
Higher bacteria, **2.18**
Hip, **5.15**
Histoplasmosis, 2.31
Histrionic personality, 7.12
HIV, **2.29**, 3.12
HLA, **1.16**
HMOs, 7.29
Hodgkin's disease, 1.29, 3.16
Homocystinuria, 4.4, 4.5
Horner's syndrome, 5.7
Howell-Jolly bodies, 1.25
HPV, 1.50
HSV, 1.50, 2.23
Humerus fracture, 5.13
Hunter syndrome, 4.13
Huntington's disease, 1.13, 1.77, 5.30
Hurler syndrome, 4.13
Hutchinson's teeth, 1.36
Hydatidiform mole, 1.54
Hydrochlorothiazide, 3.22
Hydroxysteroids, 4.28
Hyperlipidemia, **3.31, 3.32**
Hypermetropia, 6.7
Hypersensitivity, **1.6**
Hypersensitivity arteritis, 1.33
Hypersensitivity pneumonitis, 1.44
Hypertension, 1.17
Hypnagogic hallucinations, 7.6
Hypnotic drugs, **3.46**
Hypochondriasis, 7.14
Hypoglossal canal, 5.6
Hypoglossal nerve, 5.8
Hypoglycemic reaction, 3.29
Hysterical neurosis, 7.14
Ibuprofen, 3.17

ICSH, 6.37
IDDM, 1.16, 1.85
Idoxuridine, 3.9
IgA deficiency, 1.21
Immunodeficiencies, **1.21**
Impetigo, 1.88
Incidence, 7.24
India ink, 2.1
Indomethacin, 3.17
Inducers, 4.43
Infectious mononucleosis, 2.23
Inflammation, **1.1**
Inflammatory bowel disease, **1.61**
Influenza, 2.24
Inotropic drugs, **3.27**
Insulin, **3.29**, 4.39, **6.36**
Insulin receptor, 6.36
Interferon, 3.9
Internal carotid artery, 5.26
Intestinal absorption, **6.32**
Ion channels, **6.2**
IP3, 6.4
IQ tests, **7.3**
Iron, 3.4, 6.32
Iron deficiency anemia, 1.24
Ischemic heart disease, **1.37**
Isoflurane, 3.48
Isolation of affect, 7.5
Isoniazid, 1.68
Isoproterenol, 3.34
Isosorbide dinitrate, 3.23
Isotretinoin, 1.36
ITP, 1.22
Jacksonian seizures, 7.16
Janeway lesions, 1.40
Jaundice, **1.65**
Jugular foramen, 5.6
Juvenile rheumatoid arthritis, 1.16
Kala-Azar, 2.33
Kartagener's, 1.43
Kawasaki, 1.33
Keratoacanthoma, 1.87
Ketamine, 3.48
Ketoconazole, 3.10

Ketogenic, 4.2
Ketosteroids, 4.28
Key enzymes, **4.25, 4.26, 4.27**
Klebsiella, 2.13
Knee, **5.16**
Knee jerk reflex, 5.37, 6.15
Koplik's spots, 1.56
Krabbe's disease, 4.18
Kübler-Ross, 7.8
Kuru, 2.27
Kussmaul respiration, 6.20
Labetalol, 3.34
Lac-operon, 4.43
Lactobacillus, 2.11
Lactose, 4.8
Lactose intolerance, 4.9
Laryngitis, 2.6
Larynx, **5.10**
L-asparaginase, 3.16
Laxatives, **3.53**
LDL, 3.31
LE cell, 1.18
Lead, 1.89, 3.4
Lead poisoning, 4.20
Lectins, 3.13
Legal issues, **7.29**
Legionella, 2.16
Legionnaire's disease, 1.45, 3.6
Leishmania, 2.33
Leishmaniasis, 3.11
Lentiform nucleus, 5.30
Lentiviruses, 2.28
Leprosy, 2.17, 3.6
Leptospirosis, 2.19
Lesch-Nyhan syndrome, 1.14, 3.18, 4.41
Leukemias, **1.28**
Leukocytosis, 1.27
Leukoencephalopathy, 2.26
Levodopa, 3.49
Leydig cells, 1.51, **4.30**
LH, 6.37
Lidocaine, 3.26
Ligase, 4.45
Listeria, 2.11
Lithium, **3.43**

Liver abscess, 2.34
Liver cell carcinoma, **1.70**
Living will, 7.29
Lobar pneumonia, 1.45
Löffler's syndrome, 1.44
Loop diuretics, 3.22
Lorazepam, 3.45
Lovastatin, 3.32
Lower motor neuron lesions, 1.77
LSD, 3.40, 7.17
Lump jaw, 2.18
Lung tumors, **1.46**
Lung volumes, **6.19**
Lyme disease, 2.19, 3.6
Lymphocytosis, 1.27
Lymphogranuloma venereum, 1.50, 2.20
Lymphomas, **1.29**
Magnesium, 3.33, 3.53
Major depression, 7.15
Major Jones criteria, 1.42
Malabsorption, **1.62**
Malaria, **2.32**, 3.11
Malate shuttle, 4.24
Maltose, 4.8
Mandible, **5.9**
Mannitol, 3.22
MAO inhibitors, 3.2, 3.42
Maple syrup disease, 4.4, 4.5
Marfan syndrome, 1.13
Marihuana, 3.40
McArdle's disease, 4.11
McMurray's test, 5.16
Measles, 2.24
Meckel's diverticulum, 5.2
Median nerve, 5.13
Mediastinum, **5.18**
Medicaid, 7.29
Medicare, 7.29
Medulla, 5.33
Medulloblastoma, 1.76
Mefloquine, 3.11
Megaloblastic anemia, 1.24
Meig's syndrome, 1.52
Meissner's corpuscle, 6.6
Melanin, 4.3

Melanoma, 1.87
Melarsoprol, 3.11
Melatonin, 4.3
MEN, **1.86**
Ménétrier's disease, 1.58
Meningioma, 1.76
Meningitis, 2.6, 3.6
Meningococcus, 2.9
Mental Retardation, **7.3**
Meprobamate, 3.46
Mercaptopurine, 3.14
Mercury, 1.89
Merkel's disks, 6.6
Mesenteric arteries, 5.20
Mesoderm, 1.76, 5.1
Mesonephros, 5.5
Metabolism, endocrine control, **4.39**
Metachromatic leukodystrophy, 4.18
Metanephros, 5.5
Metaproterenol, 3.28, 3.34
Metastases, **1.10**
Methadone, 3.41
Methanol, 3.4
Methicillin, 3.7
Methotrexate, 3.14, 3.17
Methoxamine, 3.34
Methyl cellulose, 3.53
Methyl-DOPA, 1.68
Methylxanthines, 3.44
Methysergide, 3.21
Metoprolol, 3.34
Metronidazole, 3.11
Micelles, 4.15
Milrinone, 3.27
Mineral oil, 3.53
Miosis, 5.7
Misoprostol, 3.33
Mitral regurgitation, 1.35
Mitral stenosis, 1.35
Mitral valve prolapse, 1.35
MODY, 1.85
Molds, 2.30
Molluscum contagiosum, 2.22
Mönckeberg's arteriosclerosis, 1.32

Monoclonal gammopathy, 1.30
Monocytosis, 1.27
Mononucleosis, 2.23
Mortality, 7.24
Motion sickness, 3.47, 3.52
Motor development, **7.1**
Mouth, **1.56**
M-protein, 1.30
Mucopolysaccharidoses, 1.12, **4.13**
Müller, 5.5
Multiple myeloma, 1.30
Multiple sclerosis, 1.16, 1.78
Mumps, 2.24
Muscarinic antagonists, **3.37**
Muscarinic receptors, **6.12**
Muscle spindle, 6.15
Muscle tone, **6.15**
Muscle types, **6.16**
Muscular dystrophies, **1.75**
Myasthenia gravis, 1.4, 3.35
Mycetoma, 2.31
Mycobacteria, **2.17**, 2.3
Mycobacterium avium complex, 3.12
Mycobacterium avium intracellulare, 2.17
Mycobacterium bovis, 2.17
Mycobacterium leprae, 2 .17
Mycobacterium tuberculosis, 2.17
Mycoplasma, 2.3
Mydriasis, 5.7
Myocardial infarction, 1.37, **1.38**, 3.23
Myoclonic seizures, 3.51
Myopia, 6.7
Naloxone, 3.41
Narcissistic personality, 7.12
Narcolepsy, 1.16, 7.6, 7.16
Nasopharyngeal carcinoma, 2.23
Natriuretic factor, 6.31
Nearsightedness, 6.7
Necator, 2.37
Negative predictive value, **7.23**
Neisseria, **2.9**
Nematodes, **2.37**
Neostigmine, 3.35
Nephritic syndrome, 1.17, 1.47
Nephrotic syndrome, 1.17, 1.47

Nerve fibers, **6.5**
Neural Crest, 1.76, 5.1
Neural Tube, 1.76, 5.1
Neuroblastoma, 1.81
Neurofibroma, 1.76
Neurolept anesthesia, 3.48
Neuroleptics, **3.50**
Neuromuscular block, 3.38
Neurotransmitters, **7.9**
Neutropenia, **1.26**
Neutrophilia, 1.27
Niacin, 3.32, 4.3
Nicotine, 3.44
Nicotinic antagonists, **3.38**
Nicotinic receptors, 6.12
NIDDM, 1.85
Niemann-Pick disease, 4.18
Nifedipine, 3.23
Nifurtimox, 3.11
Night terrors, 7.6
Nitroglycerin, 3.23
Nitrous oxide, 3.48
Nocardia, 2.18
Non-Hodgkin lymphoma, 1.29, 1.7
Normal flora, **2.2**
NSAIDs, **3.17**
Nucleotides, **4.40**
Null hypothesis, 7.25
Nystagmus, **6.8**
Nystatin, 3.10
Observational cohort, **7.26**
Obsessive compulsive, 7.13
Obstructive lung disease, **1.43**
Okazaki fragments, 4.45
Oligoclonal bands, 1.78
Oligodendroblastoma, 1.76
Omeprazole, 3.33
Onchocerca, 2.37
Oncogenes, **1.7**
Oncoviruses, 2.28
Operant conditioning, 7.4
Operator, 4.43
Operon, 4.43
Opiates, 3.4, 7.17, **3.41**
Optic canal, 5.6

Oral contraceptives, 3.39
Orbital fissure, 5.6
Organophosphates, 3.4, 3.35
Orthostasis, 6.26
Osler nodes, 1.40
Osmic acid, 2.1
Osmoregulation, **6.30**
Osmotic diuretics, 3.22
Osteoarthritis, 1.71
Osteoblastoma, 1.74
Osteochondroma, 1.73
Osteogenesis imperfecta, 1.72
Osteoid osteoma, 1.74
Osteoma, 1.74
Osteomalacia, 1.72
Osteomyelitis, 3.6
Osteopetrosis, 1.72
Osteoporosis, 1.72
Osteosarcoma, 1.74
Otitis media, 2.6
Ototoxicity, 3.3
Ovarian tumors, **1.52**
Ovaries, 5.23, **4.32, 4.33**
Oxygen binding curve, **6.24**
p value, 7.25
p24, 2.29
Pacinian corpuscle, 6.6
Paget's disease, 1.55, 1.72
Pain, 1.1
Pancuronium, 3.38
Papilloma, 1.55
Papovavirus, 2.22
Paradoxical cold, 6.6
Paragonimus, 2.35
Parallel play, 7.1
Paraneoplastic syndromes, 1.46
Paranoid personality, 7.12
Parasympathetic ganglia, **5.29**
Parasympathetic nerves, 6.11
Parathyroids, **1.84**
Parietal cells, 6.33
Parkinson's disease, 1.77, **3.49**, 5.30
Parvovirus, 2.22
PAS, 2.1
Passive-aggressive personality, 7.12

Pasteurella, 2.15
Patent ductus arteriosus, 1.35, 1.36
Pedigrees, **1.11**
Pellagra, 4.4
Pelvic fractures, 5.15
Pelvic inflammatory disease, 3.6
Pemphigoid, 1.88
Pemphigus, 1.88
Penicillins, **3.7**
Pentazocine, 3.41
Peptic ulcer, **3.33**
Perfusion, 6.26
Pericarditis, **1.41**
Peripheral neuropathy, 5.35
Peripheral vascular resistance, 6.1
Peritoneum, **5.21**
Peritonitis, 5.21
Peroneal nerve, 5.17
Personality disorder personality, 7.12
Personality types, **7.12**
Pertussis toxin, 2.4
Petit mal, 3.51, 7.16
Peutz-Jeghers, 1.60
Phacomatoses, 1.13
Phagocytosis, 1.1
Pharyngeal clefts, 5.3
Pharyngeal pouches, **5.4**
Pharyngitis, 2.6, 3.6
Phencyclidine, 3.40
Phenobarbital, 3.46, 3.51
Phenothiazine, 3.50
Phenoxybenzamine, 3.34
Phentolamine, 3.34
Phenylbutazone, 3.17
Phenylephrine, 3.34
Phenylketonuria, 1.12, 4.4, 4.5
Phenytoin, 3.26, 3.51
Pheochromocytoma, 1.81
Philadelphia chromosome, 1.28
Phlebothrombosis, **1.31**
Phobia, 7.13
Phosphodiesterase inhibitors, 3.27, 6.4
Phospholipids, **4.16**
Photosensitivity, 3.3, 4.20

Physical abuse, 7.18
Physostigmine, 3.35
Piaget, 7.2
Pick's disease, 1.77
Picorna virus, 2.24
Pilocarpine, 3.36
Pindolol, 3.34
Pirenzepine, 3.33
Pituitary, **1.79**, **1.80**
Pityriasis, 1.88
Placenta, **1.54**
Plague, 2.15, 3.6
Plasma cell neoplasia, **1.30**
Platelet aggregation inhibitors, **3.24**
Play, 7.1
Plummer's disease, 1.82
Plummer-Vinson syndrome, 1.24
Pneumoconiosis, 1.44
Pneumocystis carinii, 2.33, 3.12
Pneumonia, **1.45**, 2.6, 3.6
Pneumotaxic center, 6.20
Poliomyelitis, 2.24
Polyarteritis nodosa, 1.33
Polycystic renal disease, 1.12, 1.13
Polymerase, 4.44
Polyposis, 1.13, **1.60**
Polysaccharides, **4.8**
Pompe's disease, 4.11
Pons, 5.27, **5.34**, **5.35**
Porcelain Gallbladder, 1.63
Porphyrias, **4.20**
Portocaval shunts, 5.20
Port-wine stain, 1.88
Positive predictive value, **7.22**
Post transfusion hepatitis, 2.6
Posttraumatic stress disorder, 7.13
Potassium sparing diuretics, 3.22
Power of attorney, 7.29
Pox, 2.22
Prader Willi syndrome, 1.15
Pralidoxime, 3.35
Prazosin, 3.34
Preload, 6.14
Presbyopia, 6.7

Prevalence, 7.24
Primaquine, 3.11
Primary biliary cirrhosis, 1.4
Primase, 4.45
Primer, 4.45
Prinzmetal's angina, 1.37
Prions, **2.27**
Probenecid, 3.18
Procainamide, 3.26
Progesterones, 3.39
Projection, 7.5
Promoter, 4.43
Pronation, 5.14
Pronephros, 5.5
Propanolol, 3.26, 3.34
Properdin, 1.3
Propoxyphene, 3.41
Prostacyclin, 3.24
Protease inhibitors, 3.12
Proteoglycans, 4.13
Proteus, 1.49, 2.13
Proton pump inhibitors, 3.33
Protozoa, **2.33**, **2.34**
Prussian blue, 2.1
PSA, 1.9
Pseudomembranous Colitis, 2.11
Pseudomonas, 2.16
Psoriatic arthritis, 1.71
Psychological development, **7.2**
Psychomotor seizures, 7.16
Psychoses, **7.15**
Psyllium seeds, 3.53
Ptosis, 5.7
Pulmonary hemosiderosis, 1.44
Pulsus paradoxus, 1.41
Purine, 4.40, **4.41**
Purine analogs, 3.14
Puromycin, 3.13
Putamen, 5.27
Pyranose, 4.6
Pyrimethamine, 3.11, 3.14
Pyrimidine, 4.40, **4.42**
Pyrimidine analogs, 3.14
Q fever, 2.21
Quinidine, 3.26

Quinine, 3.11
Radial nerve, 5.13
Randomized clinical trials, **7.25**
Ranitidine, 3.33
Rationalization, 7.5
Raynaud's phenomenon, 1.23
Reaction formation, 7.5
Recurrent nerve, 5.10
Red blood cells, **1.25**
Red muscle, 6.16
Reducing sugars, 4.6
Reed-Sternberg cells, 1.29
Refractory phase, 6.2
Regression, 7.5
Regulator gene, 4.43
Reiter's syndrome, 1.16
Relapsing fever, 2.19
REM sleep, 7.6
Renal blood flow, 6.29
Renal osteodystrophy, 1.84
Renal toxicity, 3.3
Renal transport, 6.28
Renin, **6.31**
Replication, **4.45**
Replication, inhibitors of, **3.14**
Repression, 7.5
Repressor, 4.43
Reserpine, 3.34
Respiratory quotient, **6.21**
Restrictive lung diseases, **1.44**
Reticulocytes, 1.25
Retinoblastoma, 1.8, 1.15
Retroperitoneum, 5.21
Retroviruses, **2.28**
Reverse transcriptase, 2.29
Reye's syndrome, 3.17
Rheumatic heart disease, **1.42**
Rheumatoid arthritis, 1.4, 1.16, 1.71
Ribavirin, 3.9
Rickettsia, **2.21**
Riedel's struma, 1.82
Rifampicin, 3.15
Rinne test, 6.10
River blindness, 2.37

RNA viruses, **2.24**
Rocky Mountain spotted fever, 2.21
Rosacea, 1.88
Roseola, 2.23
Rotator cuff, 5.11
Rotavirus, 2.24
Roth spots, 1.40
Rotor syndrome, 1.65
Roundworms, 2.37
Rubella, 2.24
Rubeola, 2.24
Saccharide, **4.8**
Saccharide disorders, **4.9**
Salicylate intoxication, 3.17, 6.22
Salmon patches, 1.88
Salmonella, 2.13
Salt retention, 4.38
Salt wasting, 4.37
Saralasin, 3.20
Scapular winging, 5.11
Scheie syndrome, 4.13
Schilder's disease, 1.78
Schistosoma mansoni, 2.35
Schizoid personality, 7.12
Schizophrenia, 7.15
Schwannoma, 1.76
Scopolamine, 3.37
Scrapie, 2.27
Seborrheic keratosis, 1.87
Secretin, 6.34
Seminoma, 1.51
Senna, 3.53
Sensitivity, **7.20**
Separation anxiety, 7.1
Sepsis, 2.6, 3.6
Sertoli cells, 1.51
Serum sickness, 1.6
Sex hormones, **3.39**
Sexual abuse, 7.18
Sheehan's syndrome, 1.80
Shigella, 2.13
Shingles, 2.23
Shoulder, **5.11**
Sick euthyroid, 1.82
Sickle cell anemia, 1.12, 1.23, 6.23

Side effects, **3.3**
Siderocytes, 1.25
Sigma factor, 4.44
Signal transduction, **6.4**
Sinusitis, 2.6
Sjögren's syndrome, **1.20**
Skeletal muscle, **6.17**
Skin cancer, **1.87**
Skin diseases, **1.88**
Skin infections, 3.10
Skull, **5.6**
SLE, 1.4, 1.16, **1.18**
Sleep apnea, 7.6
Sleep stages, **7.6**
Sleep walking, 7.6
Sleeping sickness, 2.33, 3.11
Slow viral diseases, **2.26**
Smallpox, 2.22, 2.23
Smooth muscle, **6.17**
Somatoform disorders, **7.14**
Somatostatin, 6.34
Somites, 5.1
Specificity, **7.21**
Spermatic cord, **5.22**
Spherocytosis, 1.13, 1.23
Sphingolipidoses, 1.12, **4.18**
Sphingolipids, **4.17**
Spikes, EEG, 7.16
Spinal shock, 3.36
Spirochetes, **2.19**
Spironolactone, 3.22
Splitting, 7.5
Spores, 2.3, 2.30
Sporotrichosis, 2.31
Sporozoites, 2.32
Spotted fever, 3.6
Squamous cell carcinoma, 1.87
St. Louis encephalitis, 2.25
Stains, **2.1**
Stanford Binet, 7.3
Staphylococci, **2.7**
Staphylococcus aureus, 2.7
Staphylococcus epidermidis, 2.7
Staphylococcus saprophyticus, 2.7

Starch, 4.8
Statistics, **7.19**
Status epilepticus, 3.51
Steroids, **4.28**
Stibogluconate, 3.11
Still's disease, 1.71
Stomach, **6.33**
Stool softeners, 3.53
Stranger anxiety, 7.1
Strawberry gallbladder, 1.63
Strawberry hemangiomas, 1.88
Strawberry tongue, 1.56
Strep throat, 2.8
Streptococci, **2.8**
Streptodigin, 3.15
Streptokinase, 3.25
Stretch reflex, 6.15
Striatum, 5.30
Stroke, 5.25
Strongyloides, 2.37
Student's t-test, 7.19
Sturge-Weber, 1.88
Subacromial bursa, 5.11
Subacute sclerosing panencephalitis, 2.26
Succinyl choline, 3.38
Sucralfate, 3.33
Sucrose, 4.8
Sugars, **4.6**
Suicide, **7.7**
Sulfinpyrazone, 3.24
Sulfonylureas, **3.30**
Supination, 5.14
Suramin, 3.11
Sympathetic nerves, 6.11
Syphilis, 1.50, 2.19, 3.6
Syringomyelia, 5.35
Systemic sclerosis, **1.19**
Taenia solium, 2.36
Takayasu's disease, 1.33
Tapeworms, **2.36**
Tardive dyskinesia, 3.50
Tay-Sachs disease, 4.18
Teichoic acid, 2.3
Tennis elbow, 5.14
Tensilon test, 3.35

Teratoma, 1.51
Terbutaline, 3.28, 3.34
Terfenadine, 3.47
Testes, 5.23
Testes tumors, **1.51**
Testis, **4.30**
Tetanus, 2.12
Tetanus toxin, 2.4
Tetracyclines, 3.13
Thalamus, 5.27, **5.31**
Thalassemias, 1.12, 1.23, 6.23
THC, 3.40
Theca cells, **4.32**
Theophylline, 3.28, 3.44
Thiazides, 3.19, 3.22
Thiopental, 3.46, 3.48
Thromboangiitis obliterans, 1.33
Thromboxane, 3.24
Thrush, 1.56
Thyroid, **1.82**
Thyroid tumors, **1.83**
Tibia, fractures, 5.17
Tibial nerve, 5.17
Tinea, 2.31
Tinnitus, 3.17
Tissue plasminogen activator, 3.25
Tolbutamide, 3.30
Tongue, **5.8**
Tonsillitis, 2.6
TORCH, 1.36
Touch receptors, **6.6**
Toxic hepatitis, **1.68**
Toxic shock syndrome toxin, 2.4, 2.7
Toxins, **1.89**, **2.4**
Toxoplasma gondii, 2.33, 3.12
Trachoma, 2.20
Traction diverticulum, 1.57
Transcriptase inhibitors, 3.12
Transcription, **4.44**
Transcription factor, 4.43
Transcription, inhibitors of, **3.15**
Transduction, 3.5
Transference, 7.5
Transformation, 3.5

Transient ischemic attacks, **5.26**
Translation, inhibitors of, **3.13**
Transplant rejection, 1.6
Transport, **6.3**
Trazodone, 3.42
Trematodes, **2.35**
Trench fever, 2.21
Treponema pallidum, 1.50, 2.19
Triamterene, 3.22
Triazolam, 3.45
Trichinella, 2.37
Trichomoniasis, 1.50, 2.34, 3.6
Tricyclic antidepressants, 3.2, 3.42
Triglycerides, 3.31
Trimeprazine, 3.47
Trimethoprim, 3.14
Tropical sprue, 1.62
Trousseau's sign, 1.31
Trypanosoma, 2.33
Trypsin, 4.2
TTP, 1.22
Tuberculosis, 2.17, 3.6
Tubocurarine, 3.38
Tularemia, 2.15
Tumor markers, **1.9**
Tumor suppressor genes, **1.8**
Turcot's syndrome, 1.60
Type I error, 7.25
Type II error, 7.25
Typhoid fever, 2.13, 3.6
Typhus, 2.21, 3.6
Tyramine, 3.42
Tyrosine kinase, 6.4
Ulcerative colitis, 1.16, 1.61
Ulnar nerve, 5.13
Ultimobranchial body, 5.4
Umbilical ligaments, 5.2
Undoing, 7.5
Undulating fever, 2.15
Upper motor neuron lesions, 1.77
Urachus, 5.2
Ureteric bud, 5.5
Urethritis, 2.6
Urinary tract infection, 3.6
Urogenital development, **5.5**

Urokinase, 3.25
Urolithiasis, **1.49**
Valproic acid, 3.51
Variance, 7.19
Vascular tone, 6.123
Vasodilatation, 1.1
Venereal disease, **1.50**
Ventilation, 6.19
Ventricular septal defect, 1.36
Verapamil, 3.23, 3.26
Vertebrobasilar artery, 5.26
Vertigo, 3.52
Viagra, 6.4
Vibrio cholera, 2.14
Vibrio parahaemolyticus, 2.14
Vidarabine, 3.9
Vincristine, 3.16
Vinyl chloride, 1.89
Virchow's triad, 1.31
Vitamin K deficiency, 1.22
Vitamins, **4.23**
Vitiligo, 1.88
Volume regulation, **6.30**
Von Gierke's disease, 4.11
Von Recklinghausen's disease, 1.76, 1.88
Von Willebrand disease, 1.13, 1.22
VZV, 2.23
Waldenström's, 1.30
Wallenberg syndrome, 5.32
Warfarin, 3.25
Warm antibodies, 1.23
Waterhouse-Friderichsen syndrome, 2.9
Weber test, 6.10
WEE, 2.25
Wegener's granulomatosis, 1.4, 1.33, 1.44
Weil-Felix reaction, 2.13
Wernicke, 5.24
Whipple's disease, 1.62, 3.6
Whooping cough, 2.16, 3.6
Wilms' tumor, 3.16
Wilson's disease, 1.69, 5.30
Wiskott-Aldrich syndrome, 1.14, 1.21
Wolff, 5.5
Woolsorter's disease, 2.11
Wuchereria, 2.37

Xanthoma, 1.88
X-linked recessive disorders, **1.14**
Yeasts, 2.30
Yellow fever, 2.25
Yersinia pestis, 2.15
Yolk sac, 1.51
Yolk stalk, 5.2
Zenker's diverticulum, 1.57
Ziehl Neelsen stain, 2.1
Zollinger-Ellison syndrome, 1.86, 3.33

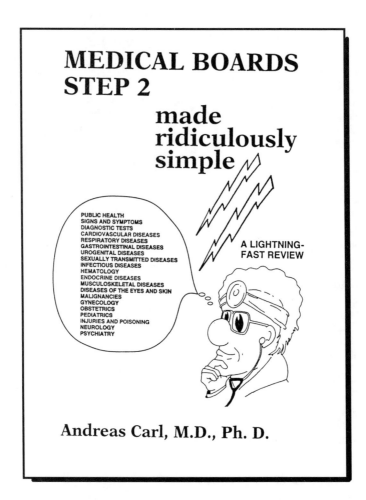

MEDICAL BOARDS STEP 2

made ridiculously simple

PUBLIC HEALTH
SIGNS AND SYMPTOMS
DIAGNOSTIC TESTS
CARDIOVASCULAR DISEASES
RESPIRATORY DISEASES
GASTROINTESTINAL DISEASES
UROGENITAL DISEASES
SEXUALLY TRANSMITTED DISEASES
INFECTIOUS DISEASES
HEMATOLOGY
ENDOCRINE DISEASES
MUSCULOSKELETAL DISEASES
DISEASES OF THE EYES AND SKIN
MALIGNANCIES
GYNECOLOGY
OBSTETRICS
PEDIATRICS
INJURIES AND POISONING
NEUROLOGY
PSYCHIATRY

A LIGHTNING-FAST REVIEW

Andreas Carl, M.D., Ph. D.

ISBN #0-940780-28-3   356 pages   273 charts $24.95

♦ All the Facts about Diseases and Organ Systems in Chart Format

♦ "Hot-Lists" cover Patient Management and Therapy

♦ In addition you should review some material from the USMLE Step 1. I recommend the following chapters from my *Medical Boards Step 1 Made Ridiculously Simple* book for "lightning fast review" of these topics:

Chapter 1 - Pathology   Chapter 2 - Microbiology   Chapter 3 - Pharmacology

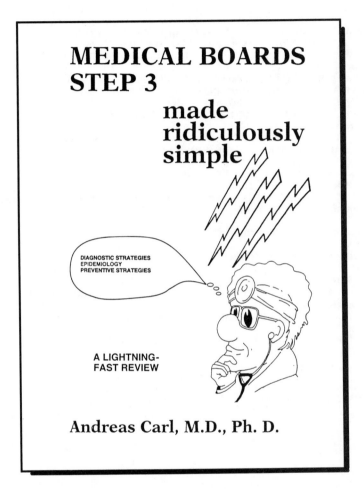

MEDICAL BOARDS STEP 3

made ridiculously simple

DIAGNOSTIC STRATEGIES
EPIDEMIOLOGY
PREVENTIVE STRATEGIES

A LIGHTNING-
FAST REVIEW

Andreas Carl, M.D., Ph. D.

ISBN #0-940780-37-2   **286 pages**   **394 charts**   **$22.95**

- Diagnostic Strategies ("what to do next ?")
- Preventive Medicine and Epidemiology of Diseases

- In addition you should review all material from the USMLE Step 2.
  I recommend my *Medical Boards Step 2 Made Ridiculously Simple* for "lightning fast review."